I0426572

My Hormones

A Simple Guide to Better and Longer Living

Mark Weis, MD

Douglas Ginter

MY HORMONES

A Simple Guide to Better and Longer Living

Copyright © 2013 by Mark Weis, MD and Douglas Ginter

All rights reserved. No part of this book may be used or reproduced in any manner whatsoever without written permission, except in the case of brief quotations embodied in critical articles or reviews. Please do not participate in or encourage the piracy of copyrighted materials in violation of the author's rights. Purchase only authorized editions.

The world as we have created it is a process of our thinking.
It cannot be changed without changing our thinking.

—Albert Einstein

"Normal" is nothing more than a cycle on a washing machine.

—Whoopi Goldberg

Table of Contents

Foreword

W elcome to the wonderful world of bioidentical hormones. We are truly blessed to live in the information era created by the Internet, a time where endless information is literally available at your fingertips. This amazing technology presents an incredible opportunity for empowering open-minded people to the possibilities for optimizing their health: gone is the paternalistic medical model where you depend solely on your physician or other healthcare providers to provide you the information they believe you need and then allowing them to make your healthcare decisions for you; arrived is today's model that allows you to seek your own information and work in collaboration with your healthcare providers to obtain the excellent health and quality of life you deserve.

However, with this freedom comes the need for caution and responsibility. The Internet and self-publishing industries create opportunities for charlatans to enrich themselves at your expense. They parade as self-anointed experts, but spout false doctrine. We urge you to exercise great care when seeking and obtaining hormone-related health and other medical information because misinformation is everywhere: on the Internet, television, radio, and other advertising mediums.

The goal of this book is to provide you a simple and easy to understand guide to bioidentical hormone replacement therapy, the medical conditions for which they are used, and they ways they can be used to help you achieve your health and wellness goals. For a simple self-assessment test, visit: ***www.myhormones.com***.

1

Meet The Clockers
Part 1: Charles

C harles Clocker is a 44 year-old male salesman at Acme Agricultural Supply in a small town in rural Indiana. He and his wife, Cindy Clocker, have been married for twenty-two years and have two children, an aging hunting dog named Rascal, and ten years remaining on the mortgage of their suburban home.

However, while all may appear rosy on the outside, things are not as they seem. Sadly, the Clocker's dog, Rascal, is depressed. Why? Because her lord and master—the aforementioned Mr. Clocker—has seemingly forgotten her. He no longer takes her on the daily walks they once enjoyed and he has skipped the last two hunting seasons, choosing instead to sit on the couch and watch football games while drinking a slowly escalating amount of beer. Rascal is deep in the throes of despair because her reasons for rising from her LL Bean doggy bed every day are gone. Why is this? She racks her canine brain, but cannot think of what she did to cause her best friend, Charles, to abandon her.

The answer, dear Rascal, is hormones—specifically lack thereof—and you can rest assured it has nothing to do with you. Charles is suffering from hormone imbalance and it is not only affecting Rascal's life; it is having serious effects on the rest of the family—potentially serious effects that could destroy the Clocker family.

Fortunately, Rascal isn't the only member of the Clocker family to have noticed Charles' behavior changes. Three months ago, after Charles' wife, Cindy Clocker, held a clandestine evening meeting in the garage with the Clocker children, the decision was made to confront Charles and get to the bottom of the situation. The following discussion occurred the next morning at the breakfast table.

Cindy (Cheerily.): "Good morning, dear. How are you feeling this morning? I made your favorite: bacon, eggs and toast with freshly squeezed orange juice."

Charles (Appearing grumpy and distracted): "Mmmm. Thanks."

Chester (12 year-old son): "Any big plans at work today, Dad? Making any big presentations? Hey—two Fridays from now is *Show Off Your Parent Day* at school. I want to bring you. Can you come?"

Charles (Mumbling, avoiding eye contact with son and rest of family.): "I don't know, C. I've got lots going on at work right now. Why don't you take your mom? She's much more interesting than me. I'm just another salesman; there's nothing special about me."

Charlotte (10 year-old daughter, emotional and barely restraining tears): "Daddy, you know that's not true! Why would you say such a thing? You and what you do are very interesting and important. I think it's mean that you won't let Chester show you off! I—"

Cindy cuts off the now sobbing Charlotte: "Charles. (No response, so raises voice). Charles! Please look at me!"

Charles raises his head wearily.

Cindy: "Charles, the children and I are worried about you. Something's not right, and we need to figure out what it is. I hope this doesn't upset you, but I made an appointment for you with Dr. Anderson at 10:00 this morning. I called your work and told them you were sick and wouldn't be coming in today."

Charles (Plaintive): "But—"

Cindy (Caring, but assertive): "No 'buts', Charles. Whatever this is, it has gone on long enough! For the past two years the children and I have watched you go from a strong, loving and wonderful man to a sad, irritable and mopey beast that is nearly impossible to live with. I know that you are a good person, and also know you can't be doing this on purpose. It's time to put an end to it! I want my husband back, and the children both want and miss their father. We leave for Dr. Anderson's office at 9:45. Be ready."

During their appointment with Dr. Anderson, the kindly physician asks Charles to describe the problems he has been experiencing that caused Mrs. Clocker to make the appointment. Charles, as per his new usual is withdrawn, quiet, and unhelpful. The physician petitions Mrs. Clocker for help and she responds that for about two years her husband has been depressed, irritable with both her and the children, basically stopped or resists participating in any marital or family activities, quit exercising and become a sluggish couch potato, is drinking more alcohol than he used to, has not gone hunting with his friends for the past two years, gained weight and, with an apologetic look towards Charles, admits that their sex life has basically died to a combination of his inability to perform sexually and lack of desire to even try. By the time she finishes relating this sobering list to the physician Mrs. Clocker's face is stained with tears.

Her worrisome description of Charles Clocker's deterioration completed, Mrs. Clocker is surprised to see Dr. Anderson's face light up, and even more shocked when he enthusiastically declares there is nothing to worry about because it's obvious that Charles has developed a classic case of major depression and treatment with an antidepressant should have him back to his wonderful previous self within a few months. He quickly scribbles a prescription for a leading antidepressant, pats Charles reassuringly on the back, and says he will see them back in one month to check on Charles' progress. Amazing, Cindy Clocker thinks to herself as she and Charles head to the parking lot! All it took was a simple fifteen minute appointment and that wonderful man divined both the mystery and the cure! Giddy with encouragement, her last thought before she slides into the passenger seat for the drive to the pharmacy is *Thank the Lord for doctors like Dr. Anderson, I'll have the old Charles back in no time!*

Oh, if only it were so. There was an itty bitty problem with what occurred during the appointment with the physician. Just because something is yellow, quacks, swims well, and its favorite food is Purina Duck Chow doesn't necessarily guarantee that the animal in question is a duck. Physicians are well aware that many diseases and medical conditions masquerade as other medical conditions. Unfortunately, our friend Charles received the wrong diagnosis from his well-intentioned family doctor and was thus prescribed the wrong treatment. As you can guess, this errant treatment will not make him better. As a matter of fact, if Charles doesn't receive the correct diagnosis soon, it's quite possible he may end up a middle-aged man who—instead of the successful salesman, husband and father he was two years ago—is unemployed, divorced, has a drinking problem, and considering suicide.

Why subject you to this depressing tale of woe? Because first and foremost this book is designed to improve your and others' lives. And also because the above scenario plays out multiple times every day in medical offices around the world, resulting in desperate people suffering from hormone imbalances that could be helped who are not helped because of the unfortunate state of ignorance among both medical professionals and lay persons regarding the importance of hormones and health.

Why does this state of ignorance exist and what can be done to correct it? This is an important question we'll address later. Let's leave poor Charles for now and discuss hormones and why they are so important.

2

Hormone Basics

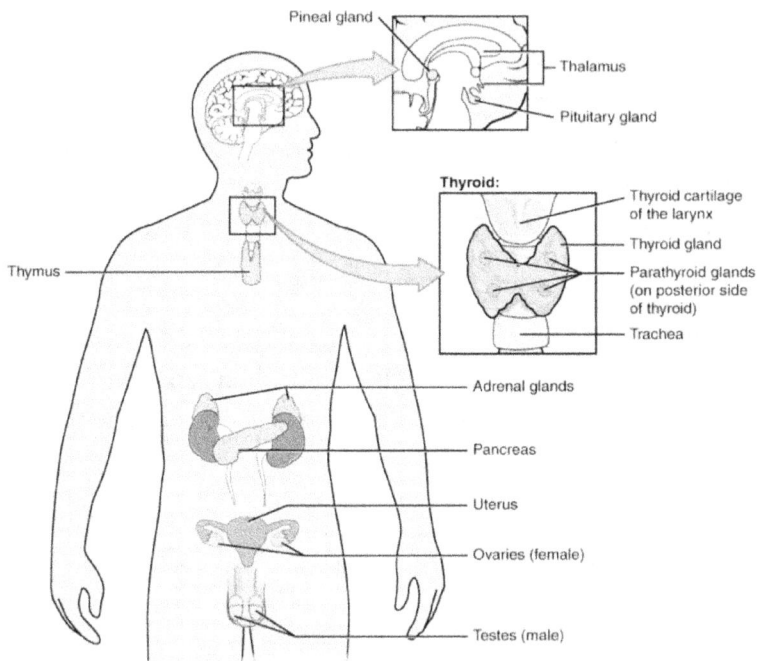

H ormones are everything. Hormone balance generally results in healthy people living long, successful, and productive lives. Hormone imbalance usually yields the opposite. Without hormone balance the human body does not work correctly, and the longer the imbalance exists the more destructive it is.. Without proper hormone function humans cannot:

- Procreate
- Think
- Eat
- Breathe
- Walk
- Talk
- Live
- And a bunch of other important things!

Now that I have your attention, and before we begin our discussion of how understanding hormones can improve your life, let's review some hormone basics.

<u>Question</u>: What is a hormone?

<u>Answer</u>: A hormone is a chemical messenger, or physiologic signal, that is produced by a gland and then sent from that gland to another organ/gland/body part to cause an action.

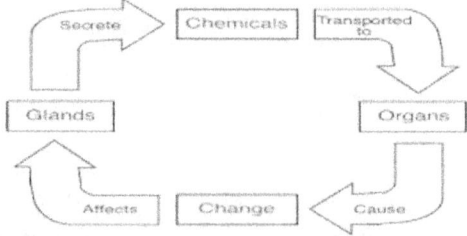

To make sure you understand what hormones are and what they do, let's examine a simple, three-step scenario:

(1) <u>Step 1</u>: ***Gland*** is assigned the task of relaying a

(2) <u>Step 2</u>: Message via a ***Hormone*** to Target Organ/Cells that orders Target Organ/Cells to perform an

(3) <u>Step 3</u>: ***Action***

Let's add biological names to this generic outline to make it into a real-life scenario:

(1) <u>Step 1</u>: Ovary (***Gland***) is assigned the task of helping regulate reproduction and menstruation so produces, then releases estrogen (hormone) which carries its

(2) <u>Step 2</u>: Message via the ***Hormone*** (estrogen) which arrives at the uterus (Target Gland/Cell), resulting in the

(3) <u>Step 3</u>: ***Action*** where the Target Organ/Cells (uterus) responds to estrogen stimulation by thickening its lining in preparation for possible embryo implantation

Another example with which you may be familiar is the role of the hormone, *insulin*, in blood sugar regulation. In this example cells in the pancreas release insulin into the bloodstream when the body detects rising blood sugar levels that occur after eating or drinking. The actions of this hormone, insulin, lower blood sugar back to normal levels, thus maintaining blood sugar balance. People that cannot produce enough insulin to maintain normal blood sugar levels suffer from a condition known as *diabetes*.

<u>Question</u>: What does *hormone balance* mean?

11

Answer: *Hormone balance* means that the amount of a hormone in your body remains at levels that allow you to function properly. Translated, your hormones are in balance if their measured levels are both:

1. At or near recommended levels <u>and</u>

2. You are not experiencing physical or mental symptoms consistent with their being too high or low.

Thus, *hormone imbalance* means the levels of a hormone in question are NOT at or near recommended levels AND you ARE experiencing physical or mental symptoms consistent with their being too high or too low.

<u>Example of hormone balance</u>: When Patient A gets his blood drawn, the laboratory reports that his IGF-1 level (test used to monitor growth hormone levels) is 175, with levels between 100 and 200 considered normal. Person A demonstrates no evidence of skin wrinkling, fatigue, muscle loss, osteoporosis, hair loss, low energy, depression, or anxiety. Because Patient A has no symptoms of growth hormone imbalance and his growth hormone levels are normal, he does not have growth hormone imbalance.

<u>Example of hormone imbalance</u>: When Patient B gets his blood drawn, the laboratory reports that his IGF-1 level (growth hormone test) is 95, with levels between 100 and 200 considered normal. Person B suffers from chronic fatigue and weakness, moodiness, low self-esteem, muscle loss, and decreased overall strength. Because Patient B does have symptoms of growth hormone deficiency and also has low growth hormone levels, he does suffer from growth hormone imbalance (deficiency).

<u>Question</u>: What are the names of the hormones you need to know?

<u>Answer</u>: We'll start with "The Big Three" because these hormones, which are classified as *sex hormones* because of their important roles in differentiation of the sexes and sexual function, receive the most press. Imbalances in any of them can wreak havoc in a person's life and on their health.

Progesterone plays important roles in menstruation, pregnancy, balancing the effects of estrogen, preventing osteoporosis and heart disease, and production of many other hormones. It is produced by the ovaries during ovulation, the adrenal glands, and nerve cells.

Estrogen is progesterone's counterpart, playing important roles in menstruation, pregnancy, balancing progesterone effects, bone growth, brain function, and development of female sex characteristics such as breasts, hips, high-pitched voice, smooth skin, and the female genitalia. The largest source of estrogen production is the ovaries, but smaller amounts are produced by the breasts, adrenal glands, and liver. An additional source of estrogen is conversion of excess testosterone to estrogen.

Testosterone plays very important roles in both men and women. Many women are shocked to discover that it is testosterone—a hormone most people associate exclusively with men—that is responsible for female sex drive! Testosterone also plays a role in women's bone health. Testosterone, scientifically classified as an *androgen* because it is essentially a male hormone and can cause *masculinization*, or body changes in women usually associated with being male such as increased body and facial hair, deepening of voice, thickening of the bones, increased musculature, and thinning hair, plays a diverse role in men analogous to the combined roles of estrogen and progesterone. It's responsible for development of male genitalia and male sexual differentiation including deep voice, thick muscles, body hair, bone growth, aggressive and assertive male behavior, libido (sex drive) and sperm production by the testes. Produced by the testes and adrenal glands in males, testosterone is also produced in small amounts by the ovaries and adrenal glands in females.

Thyroid Hormone is produced by the thyroid gland and plays critical roles in many body processes, including regulation of metabolism, energy, weight, cardiac (heart) function, behavior and mood, skin, hair, cognition (thinking, memory and mental processes), libido, reproduction, protein regulation, helping other hormones function correctly, and numerous other body processes. Because thyroid hormone plays an integral role in general body *homeostasis* (physiologic stability) and proper function of other hormones, abnormalities of thyroid hormone balance can result in medical problems ranging from mild to fatal. Prompt recognition and treatment of imbalances of this vital hormone are a must for anyone seeking hormone balance and optimal health and wellness.

Dehydroepiandrosterone, more commonly known as ***DHEA***, is involved in the production of the sex hormones by functioning as an intermediate, or *precursor*, of testosterone, estrogen and progesterone. Because all three of these hormones are derived from DHEA, which is produced in the gonads, adrenal glands, and brain, imbalances in this hormone can potentially result in imbalances in all of the sex hormones. DHEA is also important in the production of cortisol.

Adrenocorticotropic Hormone, also known as *ACTH*, like thyroid hormone, plays an integral role in overall human wellness. Although ACTH is not as well-known by the lay community as other hormones described here, the importance of ACTH imbalance and the devastating effects this condition can have on health and wellness have long been appreciated by the mainstream medical community. The role of ACTH, a hormone produced by the anterior pituitary gland in the brain, the *gonads* (testes in men, ovaries in women), and the adrenal glands is to regulate *cortisol* production and release by the adrenal glands to help manage mental and physical stress. Chronically low levels of ACTH can result in *Addison's disease*, also known as chronic adrenal insufficiency, a devastating condition that results in numerous severe symptoms and often leads to premature death.

Cortisol is a hormone produced by the adrenal glands in response to stress. Its primary functions include raising blood sugar, reducing immune system activity, and regulating metabolism of fat, protein, and sugar. Cortisol imbalance has numerous significant potential consequences: Low cortisol levels resulting from unrelenting and poorly managed stress can result in *adrenal fatigue*, a debilitating condition that is becoming increasingly common in our frenetic society; severe deficiencies in cortisol production caused by adrenal gland disease result in Addison's disease; and overproduction of cortisol leads to Cushing's disease, another condition with significant negative health consequences.

Growth Hormone, also known as *somatropin*, has received a great deal of press during the past ten years because of celebrity endorsements touting its benefits in combatting a plethora of age-related conditions ranging

15

from wrinkle reduction to life prolongation. This hormone is critical to human growth and development, with deficiencies in childhood resulting in short stature and numerous other medical and social concerns. However, studies performed in the past twenty years and innumerable anecdotal (individual cases) reports resulting from worldwide use of the drug suggest that growth hormone provides a lengthy list of potential benefits on age-related concerns such as fatigue, worsening skin quality, musculature, strength, sexual performance, depression and anxiety, cognition, and overall vitality, amongst others.

3

Meet the Clockers Part II: The Rest of the Story

C harles was unimproved at his one month follow-up appointment. Dr. Anderson encouraged Charles to continue taking the antidepressant for one more month because, as is correct, it often takes two to three months to achieve maximal antidepressant effect. To "boost things along", the well-intentioned physician raised the dosage of the medication and boldly predicted that "This new dose and 30 more days will surely do the trick!"

Dr. Anderson was both surprised and disappointed to discover at Charles' two month follow-up appointment that his patient was not only unimproved, but had actually worsened since he began taking the antidepressant. Making matters even worse was Charles was now experiencing side effects from the higher dose of the medication that included nausea, dizziness and sleepiness.

Was Dr. Anderson guilty of malpractice? Was his decision to diagnose Charles with major depression and not the hormone imbalance that was the actual cause of his symptoms evidence that he is a bad doctor? The answer is no. But how can that be? Aren't doctors taught everything they need to know to get us well when we are sick and keep us healthy we are not? The unfortunate answer is that doctors cannot know what they are not taught. The reality

17

of medical education today is that doctors and other medical practitioners are taught by the mainstream medical community, with the result that the conditions they know and are able to effectively treat are limited to the opinions of their very conservative teachers, the curriculums they institute, and the medical governing organizations overseeing them that dictate what is appropriate and acceptable, and what is not.

So how does Charles' story end? Let's review a symptom comparison of the diagnosis he was given by his physician and the diagnosis from which he actually suffered.

Major depression	Andropause (low testosterone syndrome)
Low mood	Moodiness
Irritability	Irritability
Loss of interest in pleasurable activities	Sleep difficulties
Sleep difficulties	Night sweats
Low energy	Fatigue
Sense of fatigue	Low energy
Concentration difficulties	Concentration difficulties
Crying spells	Fuzzy thinking
Anxiety or sense of restlessness	Memory impairment
Appetite disturbance	Muscle decrease
Libido decrease	Stamina decrease
Sexual difficulties	Erectile dysfunction
Memory disturbance	Decreased libido
Weight gain or weight loss	Depression
Inappropriate sense of guilt	Anxiety
Indecisiveness	Weight gain
Unexplained physical symptoms	Breast enlargement
Feelings of worthlessness	Thinning hair
Thoughts of suicide	Sleep apnea
Decreased self-esteem	Decreased work performance

Hmmm...Eerie, isn't it? When you compare the two conditions side by side, Dr. Anderson no longer appears a quack simpleton. The symptoms are almost exactly the same! How could he have known whether Charles was suffering from major depression or *andropause*, whatever the heck that is?

First, you can't make the diagnosis if you don't think of it. Taking that idea a step further, if you don't know it, you can't think of it. Because Dr. Anderson went to medical school thirty years ago, participates in very few continuing medical educational activities and restricts his learning to conditions with which he is familiar and comfortable, he couldn't diagnose low testosterone syndrome because has never heard of it, and was therefore unable to help Charles.

Second, if Dr. Anderson had known about andropause—which, by the way, is the medical term for male menopause and is also known as low testosterone syndrome or *Low T*—he would have known that the way to decide whether or not Charles' symptoms were the result of Low T is by testing Charles' total testosterone and free testosterone hormone levels. If these hormone levels were both low or near low, the doctor could have literally shown Charles his problem by pointing to the piece of paper on which the laboratory findings were printed, and provided the Clockers the solution to removing the menace that had invaded and was destroying their once-happy home.

The last item in this stepwise treatment process is to treat the patient and see if they get better. Fortunately for the Clockers, their son, the enterprising young Chester C. Clocker, saw a television commercial for a condition called *Low T*. Chester was stunned as he listened to the symptoms of this dread condition that could be fixed simply by taking the miracle cure touted by the advertisement. Amazed, he realized his father had been demonstrating nearly all of those symptoms for the past couple of years! He then dashed to the Internet, spent hours becoming knowledgeable in the condition, and then invited the family to gather round the screen for a lecture on testosterone deficiency. The group agreed that this hormone imbalance provided an excellent explanation of Dad's deterioration, so Mom called Dr. Anderson's office the next morning and

19

inquired about getting Charles tested for andropause. Unfortunately, neither Dr. Anderson nor his nurse had ever heard of such a condition so they recommended he see a doctor who specialized in hormone problems. Three months later, Charles was much improved and life in the Clocker home was returning to normal.

What's the message? Why tell you the Clockers' tale of misery followed by redemption thru hormone replacement therapy? Because, while the primary goal of this book is to teach you hormone basics and how bioidentical hormones can improve your health and quality of life, another goal is to spread this gospel to mainstream medicine. For every person whose health is improved by bioidentical hormone replacement therapy, many remain untreated because their healthcare provider is either unaware of the possible benefits of bioidentical hormone replacement therapy, or is afraid to learn this cutting edge information and put this knowledge into use by treating patients suffering from hormonal imbalance. Why is this? Because of their understandable and realistic fears that doing so could result in their being sanctioned by nearsighted state medical licensing boards and other regulatory agencies whose policies and rules are often based on antiquated and outdated science. These myopic organizations are quick to impose penalties on physicians and other medical providers who dare to think outside of their severely restrictive definitions of "the box".

The glorious age of bioidentical hormone replacement therapy is upon us! Each and every one of us must share the joyous news with our friends, family, colleagues and healthcare workers that correction of hormone imbalance with bioidentical hormone replacement therapy provides a unique and safe method of improving overall health and quality of life.

4

Bioidentical vs Synthetic Hormones

A s previously discussed, the goal of this book is to educate you about the potential health benefits of *bioidentical hormone replacement therapy* (we'll call this BHRT for the rest of the book) and empower you to make intelligent and well-reasoned decisions for incorporating this effective tool into your health and wellness efforts. What are *bioidentical hormones* and how do they differ from the *synthetic*, or artificial, hormones prescribed by most medical providers? That's easy! Just think about the meaning of the two components of the term *bioidentical*: "Bio" stands for "biological" and "identical" means "exactly the same". Therefore, bioidentical hormones are hormones that are exactly the same as those made by the body. Made from soy and yams, bioidentical hormones are *natural* in that they (1) come from nature and (2) are *molecularly identical*—or biologically the same—as the hormones made by our bodies, making bioidentical hormones the ideal treatment for achieving hormone balance in persons suffering from hormone deficiency syndromes and other hormone imbalance concerns.

In contrast to natural bioidentical hormones, the synthetic, or non-bioidentical, hormones created in laboratories by large pharmaceutical companies are not molecularly identical to the hormones our body makes. Why do pharmaceutical companies do this? Because the first rule of business is that in order for a business to succeed it must make enough money to pay its bills and make a profit. Pharmaceutical companies make their money and stay in business by developing *molecular compounds* (drugs) that can be patented. And only *novel* (new), or *biologically unique* (previously undiscovered), compounds can be patented. Once a compound is patented, no other company is allowed to sell that exact compound for the life of the patent, which may range from a few to many years. In order to remain competitive and stay in business, pharmaceutical companies must make large profits off the drug while their product is under patent. Why? Because when the drug's patent expires, other companies are allowed to create a *generic*, or copycat, version of that same drug and sell/compete against the company that originally created the drug. Doesn't sound fair to the drug company, does it? They do the work and then these other pirates are allowed to steal their product and sell it? Who designed that system?! But that's the way the pharmaceutical industry works. The money the original company makes off the novel compounds they discover and sell is used to run the company, pay shareholders, and finance the research and development required to create new drugs. So the reasons they design artificial, or synthetic, hormones is that they are operating according to the business realities of the pharmaceutical industry; this doesn't make them bad people, members of an evil empire, and it isn't morally wrong—it just means that most of the hormones they make aren't bioidentical, or molecularly the same as the ones our body makes, because of the catch 22 that they can't patent bioidentical hormones because they already exist and so don't qualify as being a "novel compound". And because of this, the synthetic, or artificial, hormones they create not only do not work as well, the fact that they differ chemically from the hormones in our bodies creates numerous potential problems that range from mild side effects to serious conditions such as increased risks for heart attacks, strokes and some cancers.

ILLUSTRATION OF BIOIDENTICAL VS SYNTHETIC HORMONE

Testosterone

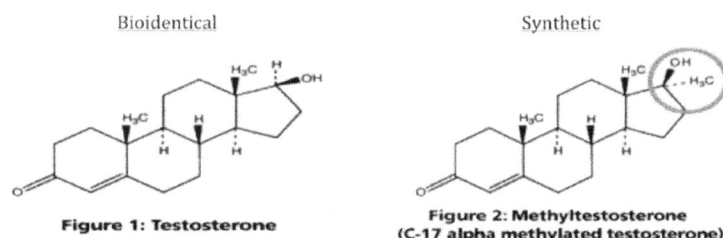

Bioidentical   Synthetic

Figure 1: Testosterone

Figure 2: Methyltestosterone
(C-17 alpha methylated testosterone)

Do you see how the area of the molecule inside the red circle in the compound on the <u>right</u> side (synthetic compound) differs from the same area in the upper right hand of the compound on the <u>left</u> side (bioidentical compound)? The testosterone molecule on the left is molecularly identical to, or exactly the same as, the testosterone produced by our bodies. Why is the fact that these two hormones differ in composition by only a couple of atoms such a big deal? The answer is that the lock-and-key mechanism hormones require to cause their biological actions requires the messenger molecule, or hormone, to be the exact one the target organ is expecting to see. If it is not, the desired action will not occur. Difference in as little as a single atom can make our body unable to recognize the molecule for what it was intended to be, creating undesired possibilities of side effects and disease.

What is this lock-and-key mechanism hormones require? In order for hormones to successfully deliver their chemical message, and for this message to cause the desired action (i.e., rising estrogen levels in a teenage female resulting in onset of puberty), the hormone must "lock" into specific receptors on

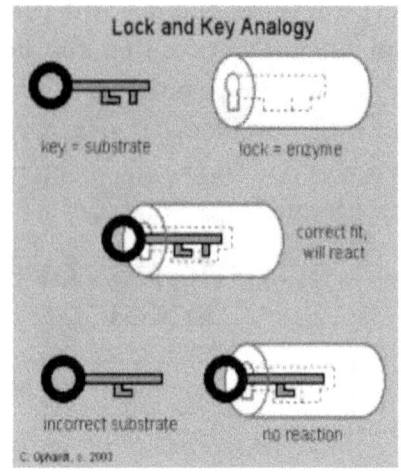

the target organ cells. In the illustration on the right, envision the hormone as the key and the receiving organ cell as the lock. If the key fits, the desired chemical reaction will occur; if it does not, the reaction will not occur and the unrecognized molecule remains in the body and will either be cleared away, or may interact with the target cell or other cells in unpredictable or possibly harmful ways. A twist on a statement from an infamous court case may help you understand the importance of the lock and key aspect of delivery of hormonal messages: "If the molecule does not fit, the target cell cannot benefit."

Before moving onto a discussion of hormone imbalances and the various medical conditions and symptoms they can cause, let's answer a couple of commonly heard questions regarding bioidentical hormones.

1. If bioidentical hormones are natural and are made from plants—specifically yams and soy—shouldn't increasing my dietary intake of those two items result in hormone balance? Good question, but the answer

is no. While bioidentical hormones are made from these two plant sources, the actual hormones themselves do not exist in the plants. Bioidentical hormones are created in laboratories from a substance present in both yams and soybeans called *diosgenin*.

2. Does it matter if the bioidentical hormone used is made from yams or soy? No. Both work equally well although most bioidentical hormones produced today originate from soy sources due to low soybean prices.

Are you wondering if your hormones may be imbalanced? The list of possible causes of hormone imbalance is very long and includes poor diet, lack of exercise, being overweight or underweight, stress, etc., but other major causes are the foods we eat and the environment we live in.

Most of the meat, poultry, and dairy products we consume are tainted with hormones. This occurs because we now live in an age where industrial farming is king, which means quality is sacrificed for quantity. The majority of our country's farms, which at one time were run by families who took pride in providing safe, high quality products, are now owned and managed by large corporations whose missions are to maximize profits, which means squeezing every last dollar out of every acre or animal. How do they do this? Through science, of course!

Tainted meat and dairy products result from the addition of hormones and antibiotics to livestock feed, and pesticides cause the fruits, vegetables, breads and other grain products on our store shelves to be contaminated with harmful chemicals. Hormones facilitate growth which leads to larger animals, and antibiotics reduce or prevent the infections that kill or inhibit stock growth. Obviously, it makes perfect sense for these new-age farmers to engage in this business improvement process because it results in greater numbers of larger animals. Unfortunately, although it's good for the farmers, it's bad for the rest of us. This is because the chemicals (hormones and antibiotics) the animals ingest, and the pesticides which the plant products are exposed to, do not "do their job and harmlessly move on". Rather, these chemicals remain in the various food products and we ingest them when we consume them, meaning that every bite of these food products may literally be poisoned with chemicals and other products that can adversely affect your health.

Added to these food-related nutrition concerns in our modern society are the toxins present in our homes, workplaces and the environment. These include *xenoestrogens* (chemicals that confuse our bodies and contribute to estrogen:progesterone imbalance by masquerading as estrogen), plastics, solvents, and other items such as PCBs.

Is there a solution to this frightening situation? Yes and no. While there is no way to live in our modern society and totally avoid all of these potential health concerns, you can dramatically reduce your exposure by:

- Staying away from processed meats like bacon, hot dogs, and sausage. They contain nitrosamines, which can lead to cancer.

- Choosing low-mercury fish like tilapia raised on American farms or branzini (European sea bass) instead of swordfish or tuna. Mercury exposure can cause memory problems, fatigue, and other health issues.

- Minimize canned food, because cans are often lined with bisphenol-A, an organic compound associated with diabetes and heart disease.

- Reduce your intake of meat and dairy products because they may contain harmful contaminants such as polybrominated diphenyl ethers, polychlorinated biphenyl, and dioxins.

- Eliminate diet soda and artificial sweeteners. Prolonged aspartame exposure can cause nerve cell damage, dizziness, and headaches.

- Be careful with farmed fish because studies show they usually contain more polychlorinated biphenyl and dramatically higher levels of dioxin than their "free range" counterparts.

- When eating chicken, choose free range (organic). Most chickens raised in industrial settings contain antibiotic resistant bacteria and *arsenic*, a chemical that can cause cancer, diabetes, and heart disease.

- Drink milk that says "no rBGH" on the carton. rBGH, or *recombinant bovine growth hormone*, has been linked with breast cancer. Other options include unsweetened soy, nut or rice milk.

- Avoid manufactured snacks. They are not only loaded with salt, corn syrup (read "sugar") and other harmful ingredients, they contain hydrogenated oils that lengthen the shelf life of the product, but will likely reduce yours because these oils are associated with diabetes and heart disease.

- Stay away from artificially-colored foods because laboratory animals exposed to these synthetic additives demonstrate increased rates of cancer.

- When buying produce, go organic. Pesticides can cause numerous health concerns, including nervous and reproductive system damage, and cancer.

- Old school is the best rule for cooking. Teflon used to create nonstick surfaces can release noxious gases when exposed to high temperatures, which puts you at risk for heart disease. Use stainless steel or cast iron cookware.

- Never microwave food in plastic bowls, containers, or dishes. Heat exposure can cause bisphenol-A found in plastics to break down and contaminate food.

5

Hormone Imbalance

*H*ormone imbalance, once considered a profane term in the halls of medicine, has become a hot phrase. And learning about it is likely one of the main reasons you chose to read this book. What is hormone imbalance and what might it mean to your health? A person suffering from hormone imbalance experiences physical or mental symptoms caused by hormone levels that are either too high or too low.

To better understand hormone balance picture a seesaw, or teeter-totter, on a playground, and then envision *hormone balance* as the state achieved when both ends of the piece of equipment are near equilibrium (horizontal). As long as both ends stay in or near this position, the piece of equipment is in balance. When one end dips down and causes the other end to rise up, the device is now out of balance and becomes unstable.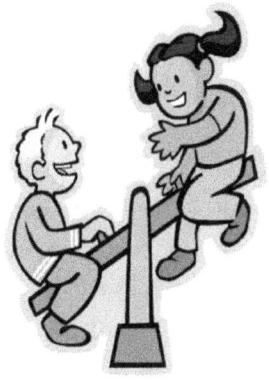

The same goes for hormones and people. When you test your hormone levels and find them to be "within normal" or "in range", you are considered to be in hormone balance if you also do not have symptoms consistent with a specific hormone imbalance. However, if your tests demonstrate that your hormone levels are either low or near low, or high or near high AND you are experiencing symptoms as a result of these abnormal hormone levels, you are "out of balance", or suffering from a hormone imbalance. As my Great Uncle Herkimer used to say, when you're imbalanced you're "out of sorts and discombobulated." And, unfortunately, discombobulated in this context can mean miserable, sick or dead.

In order to better under understand hormone imbalance and how it might relate to your health, here are a couple more definitions and suggestions regarding HRT.

Hormone Imbalances Present As Syndromes

In general, an imbalance of a hormone—whether that hormone level is too high or too low—is unlikely to manifest as a single physical or mental effect (*symptom*), but is more likely to present as a group of symptoms that healthcare professionals call *syndromes*. One example of a syndrome would be a person with an underactive thyroid gland that results in low levels of thyroid hormone. This condition is called *hypothyroidism*, and people with hypothyroidism rarely experience only a single symptom such as fatigue. They are more likely to suffer from a cluster of symptoms (syndrome) such as fatigue, weight gain, depression, cold intolerance and constipation. Another example would be *premenstrual syndrome*, a syndrome cause by a relative deficiency of the hormone progesterone in relationship to the hormone estrogen. This condition is not associated with a single problem such as abdominal cramps, but is usually characterized by many of the following symptoms, including bloating and water retention with resulting weight gain, breast tenderness and lumpiness, headaches, cramps, fatigue, irritability, mood swings, and anxiety.

Abnormal Hormone Levels By Themselves May Not Require Hormone Replacement Therapy

Just because laboratory tests show that one or more of your hormone levels is high or low does not mean you must start BHRT. Knowledgeable physicians and other healthcare professionals are taught to treat the patient—not the lab value, x-ray report, or other test. The decision as to whether or not BHRT may be right for you should be based on the equation:

> SYMPTOMS of a specific hormone imbalance
>
> +
>
> LABORATORY TESTS that confirm/suggest the same hormone imbalance
>
> =
>
> TREAT with BHRT

Let's look at two examples. Which of these people do you think should receive hormone replacement therapy and who should not?

1) Jane is 40 years old, her symptoms are consistent with low cortisol, and her lab tests suggest she may be suffering from cortisol deficiency, also known as *adrenal fatigue.*

2) Julie is 42 years old, feels a bit out of sorts, her lab tests show no significant hormone level abnormalities, and she is doing okay in general.

Who do we treat? Jane, of course! See, it's not that hard. To find out if you suffer from hormone imbalance go to ***www.myhormones.com*** to order a quick, painless, inexpensive and easy to use at-home saliva hormone test. If you already know you suffer from hormone imbalance, contact the professionals at Fountain of Youth MD to find a doctor that can help restore your hormones to ideal levels and return you to optimal health.

Now that you're getting the hang of it, let's spend some time learning about the specific hormone imbalances.

6

Exercise and Nutrition

O ne of the biggest complaints voiced about the US healthcare system is, instead of creating a system designed to reduce cost of healthcare by preventing medical problems the American approach is to allow illness to develop and then spend obscene amounts of money treating it. While that may be a bit harsh, it's essentially true. Many of us have lost sight of the simple truth that the ideal path to health and wellness is to avoid becoming ill, and the best method for avoiding illness is to engage in a lifestyle focused on regular exercise, proper nutrition, and minimization of stress. We have become a nation of overweight, overstressed, malnourished and physically unfit creatures that want to take a pill for everything. And unfortunately, because the rest of the world—especially its children—admire the American way of life, millions of others around the world are following suit.

The first lesson in the identification and treatment of hormone imbalance is that much of is caused, and can be reversed by proper diet, exercise, and stress reduction. Newton's Law of Motion that states "A body at rest remains at rest" applies here. Our bodies are built for movement, and if we don't continually move them they deteriorate and become inflexible. Inertia kills—it accelerates the aging process and contributes to diseases such as high blood pressure, obesity, high cholesterol, diabetes, and other risk factors for developing heart disease, stroke, cancer and other catastrophic life-shortening illnesses.

If you live a sedentary lifestyle comprised of sitting and eating and little to no exercise, your first step in addressing hormone imbalance is beginning an exercise program. As always, consult your personal physician or other healthcare provider before doing this, but once you start you should create a regimen composed of activities that you enjoy because if you don't, it's unlikely you'll stick with it. Keys to creating an exercise program you will maintain are choosing activities you enjoy such as tennis, golf, walking, swimming; having an exercise partner who will help keep you accountable (and you will keep them accountable); and varying your exercise routine. An example of varying exercise routine would be walking with a friend three days a week and playing tennis or racquetball two days a week, and going for an occasional long bike ride. Please know you don't have to engage in intense exercise that leaves you bedridden from pain for two days in order to improve your health. Easy, comfortable aerobic activity lasting 20-30 minutes is all you need. Do that five times per week on a consistent basis and you'll be on the way to better health and a longer, more satisfying life!

Paradoxically, at the same time that America's overall level of fitness has been declining, health and fitness has become a major industry. Mega-gyms are appearing on every street corner, and vitamin and supplement stores abound that tout the benefits of pills, powders, lotions and potions that burn fat, build lean muscle, and cure everything from hiccups to hemorrhoids without your having to leave the couch. Competition is fierce and promises ranging from the outrageous to the bizarre can leave you confused, suspicious, and jaded. The best advice as regards all this is to remember that anything that sounds too good to be true usually is.

Another commonly heard quotation that applies to this situation is "You are what you eat." A diet high in saturated fats (found in fatty meats, full dairy products), high in simple sugars and other non-complex carbohydrates, and low in quality protein is a recipe for poor health. Following the guidelines below should help you improve your approach to nutrition, feel better, lose weight or maintain a healthy weight, and prevent diet-related hormone imbalance and other medical concerns.

Big Picture: Eat 5-6 small meals per day instead of 2-3 large meals per day, limit fat intake to 10 to 20% of total calorie intake, drink plenty of water (at least eight glasses per day), eat complex carbohydrates and lean proteins, and limit simple sugars.

Rule 1: Avoid fatty foods (especially animal fats), excessive salt and simple sugars. This eliminates nearly all fast foods, chips, candy and soft drinks. Who needs them? Certainly not you if you wish to eat right and get in shape! Most people find that within a few weeks they no longer desire these toxic items.

Rule #2: Make time for a breakfast containing complex carbohydrates and protein. This will improve your metabolism, improve your energy levels, and provide the proper fuel for building muscle and maintaining body homeostasis. Easy to prepare examples include a quality protein shake, bowl of oatmeal, scoop of cottage cheese, fruit and coffee.

Rule #3: Eat small meals every 3 to 4 hours throughout the day and have each meal contain protein and low glycemic carbohydrates. Examples include combinations such as tuna with brown rice, lean meat with red baked potato, cottage cheese with berries, chicken with whole grain pasta, lean ground turkey with salsa, spinach and small apple, etc.

Rule #4: If you're looking to gain weight, eat larger portions and eat more frequently. If you wish to lose weight, maintain the same eating frequency but reduce portion size and consume the majority of your calories and carbohydrates in the first half of your day. Evening eating should include a source of protein and little to no carbohydrates.

Rule #5: Attempt to achieve a 50:50 balance of protein to carbohydrate intake to build and maintain a lean body.

Rule #6: Between-meal snacking is only acceptable if the snack is truly nutritious. Do not substitute snacks for meals. Acceptable snack option examples include fruits or vegetables, protein bars, whole wheat bagels, cottage cheese, and small ready to drink protein shakes.

Rule #7: Avoid simple carbohydrates. Simple carbohydrates (sugar) provide quick energy but this is usually followed by a *hypoglycemic* (low blood sugar) "crash". In addition, excessive sugar intake can lead to blood sugar problems, diabetes, weight gain, fatigue and increased fat storage. When you do eat carbohydrates, make sure to eat a protein source at the same time because this slows carbohydrate absorption, which results in decreased absorption of carbohydrate calories.

Rule #8: Fuel your body before exercising. Eat a small meal 30-60 minutes before you exercise. Having complex carbohydrates in your system should provide the energy you need to participate fully in physical activity and help prevent low blood sugar-related problems such as tremor, nausea, weakness or dizziness.

<u>Rule #9</u>: Your body's most critical nutritional requirement is water. Tissue quality, performance, resistance to injury, and waste excretion depend on adequate intake of high quality water. Drink frequently throughout the day and during exercise.

<u>Rule #10</u>: Don't forget the basics: Adequate sleep, rest and relaxation are required for a healthy body and a healthy mind.

7

Thyroid Hormone Imbalance: Hypothyroidism

When Sally married John at age twenty-five she weighed 115 pounds and wore a size 2 dress. At age forty-three Sally began gaining weight. Now forty-seven, she weighs 185 pounds and for the past few years has been suffering from depression, anxiety spells, fatigue, dry skin, and is always cold. No matter how hard she battles against her weight and other problems with diets, exercise, diet pills, fat burners, antidepressants, anti-anxiety agents and energy drinks, nothing seems to help. Today it all came crashing down on her and she officially lost hope. So when her wonderful husband John arrived home late from work, he found her sobbing on their bedroom floor sprawled amidst dozens of unflattering outfits of varying sizes she had purchased over the past few years in attempts to hide her weight gain.

Poor Sally. She, like innumerable others suffering from undiagnosed hypothyroidism, is in a bad way. And I bet her dutiful husband John is a bit more frustrated both with her and for her than he lets on. Hypothyroidism is a very common condition that causes physical and mental problems for many people. Fortunately, diagnosis and appropriate treatment of this condition usually results in improvement or elimination of many of these concerns.

Unfortunately, many people are unaware of the condition and so do not recognize the obvious symptoms of hypothyroidism even when they have been suffering from it for years. Also unfortunately, the outdated hypothyroidism laboratory testing guidelines used by most of today's mainstream physicians result in many peoples' thyroid imbalances going unrecognized and their not receiving the safe and effective treatment that would likely greatly improve their health and quality of life.

Most leading hormone self-help books contain sections describing specific hormone imbalance states. And nearly all of them spend most of their time on estrogen and progesterone. Why? Because these are the sex hormones with which women are most acquainted, and until the recent information barrage related to testosterone deficiency, women interested in improving their health purchased the lion's share of books like this one. As a result, women believe these are the hormones they should learn about, so they seek books heavy on estrogen and progesterone.

That's both good and bad. Why? It's GOOD because the reasons that women—and men for that matter—buy health improvement books are because they believe that learning about the deleterious effects of medical issues like hormone imbalance can help improve their health, their quality of life, and possibly prolong their life. And it's BAD because the list of the most common symptoms seen with hormone imbalance includes problems such as fatigue, weight gain, depression, anxiety, irritability, decreased libido, poor sexual performance, and the like. And while many of these concerns can result from imbalances in the sex hormones, estrogen and progesterone—the two hormones associated with menstrual problems and menopause; and testosterone, the hormone associated with masculinity—thyroid dysfunction is also a common and very correctable cause of many of these same issues that can wreak havoc on woman's life.

Because balanced sex hormone states are a must for good health, we'll pay great attention to them. However, the hormone imbalance section of this book begins with thyroid imbalance for five reasons:

1. Untreated thyroid imbalance is very common and much more common than most patients or healthcare providers are aware of.

2. Shockingly, many hormone imbalance self-help texts provide little to no information on thyroid imbalance.

3. Untreated thyroid imbalance impairs, and can destroy quality of life and makes people miserable.

4. Untreated thyroid imbalance increases the risk for developing many serious medical conditions, including heart attack, stroke, depression, anxiety, dementia, obesity, diabetes, and others.

5. Untreated thyroid imbalance can be fatal.

ROLE OF THYROID HORMONE

The thyroid is one of the most important organs in the human body. Located in the neck on either side of the voice box, its numerous roles include regulation of metabolism, organ and overall body growth, and helping other hormones do their jobs, among numerous other tasks. It produces two thyroid hormones: T3, or *triiodothyronine*, and T4, *thyroxine*, and also produces *calcitonin*, a hormone involved in calcium regulation.

Thyroid hormone production is regulated by two hormones produced by organs in the brain: (1) *thyrotropin releasing hormone* (TRH), which is produced by the hypothalamus, and (2) *thyroid stimulating hormone* (TSH), which is produced by the anterior pituitary gland. Thyroid production and release occurs via the following step-wise process.

<u>Step 1</u>: The *hypothalamus* releases TRH. TRH stimulates the

<u>Step 2</u>: *anterior pituitary gland* to release TSH. TSH stimulates the

<u>Step 3</u>: *thyroid gland* to release T3 and T4

<u>Step 4</u>: The *hypothalamus* determines the need to release more or less TRH by monitoring blood levels of T3 and T4 in the body. This is called a *negative feedback loop*. When the hypothalamus detects that the body's levels of thyroid hormone (T3 and T4) are too low, it increases production and release of TRH in order to raise thyroid hormone levels. When the hypothalamus detects that the body's levels of thyroid hormones are normal or too high, it withholds release of TRH.

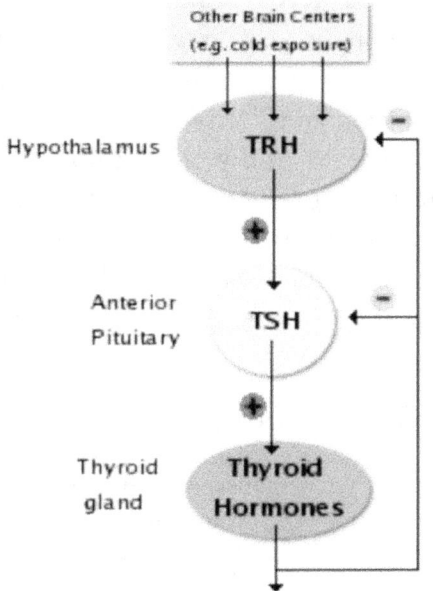

Other Brain Centers
(e.g. cold exposure)

Hypothalamus **TRH** −

⊕

Anterior
Pituitary **TSH** −

⊕

Thyroid **Thyroid**
gland **Hormones**

target cells throughout body

SYMPTOMS OF THYROID HORMONE IMBALANCE

Hypothyroidism can result in many symptoms. An easy way to remember what hypothyroidism means is to— as we did with the word *bioidentical*—break the term into its component parts. First, *hypo* means "below" or "too low"; second, *thyroidism* means "symptom complex relating to the thyroid". So, if we add *hypo* (too low) to *thyroidism* (thyroid symptom complex) the result would be a "symptom complex resulting from low levels of thyroid hormone". The trick to remembering what *hypo* means is easy: just remember there is an "O" in "hypo" and an "O" in "low", so "hypo" means "low." How low can you go?!

Continuing in the same vein, the meaning of *hyperthyroidism*, which is a "symptom complex related to high thyroid hormone levels", can be remembered the same way. *Hyper* is the opposite of *hypo*, so *hyper* means "above" or "too high". Add *hyper* (excessive) to *thyroidism* (thyroid symptom complex) and you get "symptom complex resulting from low levels of thyroid hormone". Another less politically correct way to remember what *hyper* means is to think of the children we went to school with who couldn't sit still or were interruptive that were labeled by teachers, parents and other children as "hyperactive" or "hyper", for short.

HYPOTHYROIDISM SYMPTOMS	
Fatigue	Dry, thin hair and hair loss
Weight gain	Decreased sweating
Puffy face	Infertility
Menstrual irregularity	Depression
Cold intolerance	Anxiety
Joint and muscle pain	Cognitive impairment
Constipation	Slowed metabolism
Dry skin	Slowed heart rate

CAUSES OF HYPOTHYROIDISM

There are numerous causes of hypothyroidism. The most common is an autoimmune disease called *Hashimoto's thyroiditis.* Autoimmune diseases are inflammatory conditions where your own body produces *antibodies* (immune cells) that attack and destroy your own tissue. This tissue destruction can result in medical problems affecting many organs that lead to disability, pain, poor general health, and premature death.

Another cause is hyperthyroidism treatments designed to lower high thyroid levels back to non-toxic, or normal, levels. These treatments include radioactive iodine, anti-thyroid medications, or surgery to remove the cancerous or non-cancerous areas of the thyroid causing the excess thyroid hormone production. Unfortunately, all these

44

treatments can result in permanent hypothyroidism requiring lifelong treatment with thyroid replacement in order to maintain thyroid hormone balance.

Medications can also contribute to hypothyroidism. An example would be lithium, a drug used in the treatment of psychiatric disorders.

Less common causes include congenital disease, pituitary and hypothalamic disease, and pregnancy. Detection and treatment of pregnancy-induced hypothyroidism is critical because if left untreated it increases the risk of numerous pregnancy complications that can result in serious harm to the developing fetus.

Lastly, a fairly common cause of hypothyroidism in developing countries is iodine deficiency. Fortunately, however, this is rarely encountered in the United States due to the addition of iodine to table salt.

DIAGNOSING HYPOTHYROIDISM

There are two classifications of hypothyroidism:

Overt hypothyroidism: Overt hypothyroidism is doctor-speak for ordinary hypothyroidism. "Overt" means "out in the open", so this term was adopted to signify that these sufferers' symptoms and laboratory examination findings demonstrated clear-cut hypothyroidism. Merely remember that *overt hypothyroidism* = hypothyroidism.

Subclinical hypothyroidism: This is a more subtle, yet still important type of hypothyroidism. In the past, many physicians and other healthcare providers did not recognize or treat subclinical hypothyroidism because it was their opinion that these patients' laboratory test results weren't bad enough to treat. Translated, these physicians chose, as do many still, to ignore these people even if they had symptoms and signs of hypothyroidism solely because their lab test results did not fall outside of the norms they were taught during their training. Fortunately, advances in the understanding of hypothyroidism have resulted in open-minded medical providers choosing to treat people and not restrict their decision-making to rigid lab result criteria, a paradigm shift that has led to identification and effective treatment of a great number of patients suffering from this "minor" thyroid imbalance. In addition, recent statements by high-level endocrine societies have advocated for a more liberal approach to the diagnosis and treatment of hypothyroidism—specifically as regards subclinical hypothyroidism.

Diagnosis of all hormone imbalances requires soliciting symptoms of the condition, performance of a physical examination, and laboratory testing. Among the physical findings listed in the Hypothyroidism Symptoms Table, a commonly encountered physical examination finding is *goiter* (neck swelling due to enlargement of the thyroid gland resulting from excessive TSH stimulation). Laboratory testing reveals:

- decreased thyroxine (T4)

- decreased triiodothyronine (T3)

- increased thyroid stimulating hormone (TSH)

Find out if you suffer from hormone imbalance, including your thyroid hormone levels, by going to ***www.myhormones.com*** to order a quick, painless, inexpensive and easy to use at-home blood spot test. If you already know you suffer from hormone imbalance, contact the professionals at Fountain of Youth MD to find a doctor that can help restore your hormones to ideal levels and return you to optimal health.

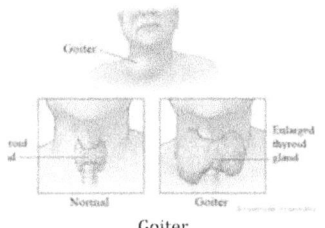

Goiter

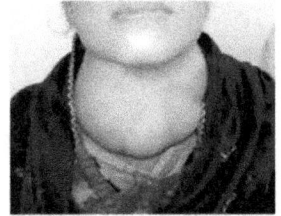

Severe goiter in Third World patient

TREATING HYPOTHYROIDISM

The treatment of most cases of hypothyroidism is fairly simple, with the majority of patients demonstrating symptom improvement within a few weeks. Treatment choices depend on the patient's specific medical situation. Knowledgeable medical providers choose to treat with a form of desiccated thyroid USP, a bioidentical product that tends to provide better clinical results than treating with T4 or T3. It is the combination of T4 and T3 and adequate levels of both of these thyroid hormones that are required to achieve thyroid balance.

8

Thyroid Imbalance: Hyperthyroidism

N ancy was worried. Over the past year she had watched helplessly as her sister's life fell apart. During this time period her sister, Alice, lost thirty pounds; received a succession of three different antidepressant and anti-anxiety combinations from her family physician in an effort to treat the severe anxiety, depression, nervousness and insomnia that began seemingly overnight; and was scheduled to see a heart specialist next week for a rapid heart rate.

What was going on? Did the weight loss mean cancer, or was her sister having a nervous breakdown? Alice had never experienced health problems before, and nothing in her life indicated a reason for her to develop mental health problems. She didn't smoke, drink alcohol, use drugs, and she exercised fairly regularly. In addition, she and her husband, Sam, had a happy marriage, both children were doing well, and their family was financially secure. Things should be fine, but they obviously weren't—not for Alice, anyway.

Enough already, she thought to herself! She was not going to stand idly by and watch her sister deteriorate into a watery pool on the floor like the Wicked Witch of the West. She sat down at the Internet, located her favorite search engine, typed in her sister's lengthy list of symptoms and then entered the phrase "medical problem". She was rewarded with page after page of results containing the terms *hyperthyroidism* and *hormone imbalance*. Hmmm…she wondered, what's hyperthyroidism? She clicked on one of the links and began reading.

SYMPTOMS OF HYPERTHYROIDISM

As previously stated, hyperthyroidism is a group of symptoms caused by high thyroid hormone levels. Like hypothyroidism, *overactive thyroid*, which is another name for hyperthyroidism, can also cause physical and mental problems that range from mild to fatal. Symptoms of hyperthyroidism include:

HYPERTHYROIDISM SYMPTOMS	
Fatigue	*Exophthalmos* (bulging eyes)
Weight loss	Sweating
Tremor	Infertility
Menstrual irregularity	Depression
Headache	Anxiety
Joint and muscle pain	Cognitive impairment
Diarrhea	Increased metabolism
Dizziness and fainting	Rapid heart rate
Memory impairment	Irritability

CAUSES OF HYPERTHYROIDISM

The most common cause of hyperthyroidism is *Grave's disease*, an autoimmune disease that affects 2% of the female population. Other, less frequently encountered causes include malignant (cancerous) and non-malignant (benign, non-cancerous) growths that produce excessive amounts of thyroid hormone.

DIAGNOSING HYPERTHYROIDISM

Diagnosing either of the thyroid imbalances—hypothyroidism or hyperthyroidism—is done in the same way. Just as with hypothyroidism, hyperthyroidism can also cause a goiter in the neck. However, the goiter seen in hyperthyroidism patients results from either inflammation-induced or cancerous swelling of the gland, as opposed to the TSH-induced thyroid gland overstimulation seen in hypothyroidism patients.

Blood or saliva testing of persons with hyperthyroidism will show:

• high thyroxine (T4)

• high triiodothyronine (T3)

• low thyroid stimulating hormone (TSH)

Find out if you suffer from hormone imbalance, including your thyroid levels, by going to ***www.myhormones.com*** to order a quick, painless, inexpensive and easy to use at-home spot blood test. If you already know you suffer from hormone imbalance, contact the professionals at Fountain of Youth MD to find a doctor that can help restore your hormones to ideal levels and return you to optimal health.

Because diagnosing hyperthyroidism usually requires additional testing, persons receiving a diagnosis of hyperthyroidism should always be referred to a hormone specialist, or *endocrinologist*. These medical specialists are trained to systematically approach the evaluation of patients suffering from hyperthyroidism in order to provide them safe and effective treatment options.

TREATING HYPERTHYROIDISM

Because of the safety concerns associated with hyperthyroidism, discussion of hyperthyroidism treatment is beyond the scope of this book. Again, everyone diagnosed with hyperthyroidism should have their case managed by an endocrinologist. However, patients with hyperthyroidism informed by their endocrinologist that part of their treatment will include thyroid replacement therapy are encouraged to ask if their hormone replacement therapy could be with bioidentical thyroid hormone.

9

Estrogen

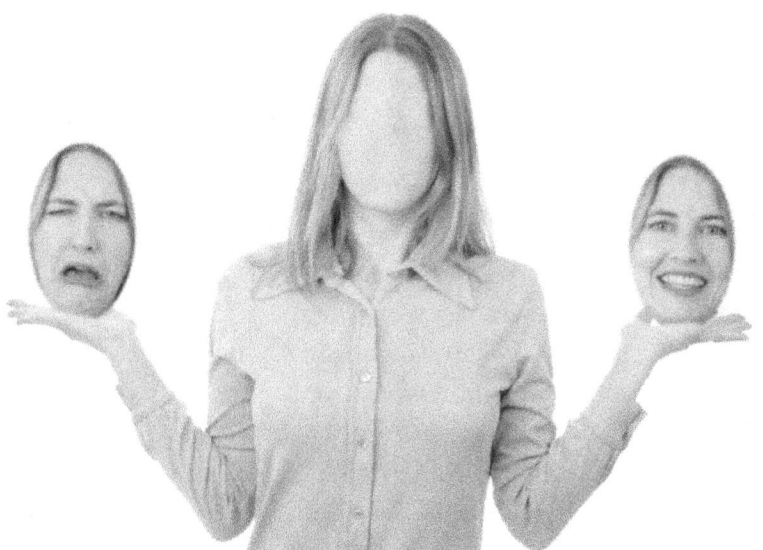

Mary couldn't take it anymore. She wiped her sweaty face and neck for the fourth time in the past hour and excused herself from the meeting—a meeting she was having great difficulty concentrating on because she was busy swinging wildly from freezing cold to burning alive. Swinging was for Tarzan and trapeze artists, and she wanted no more of it! The hot flushes, combined with the other issues she had been experiencing lately including vaginal dryness, sexual problems, breast tenderness and foggy thinking, had her at her wit's end.

Her co-worker, Thelma, had noticed her struggling and asked if anything was the matter. After hearing Mary's list of miseries, Thelma chuckled and responded that it looked like Mother Nature was doing its thing and Mary was going through "the change". Mary responded she had figured as much, and told Thelma she didn't know what to do because she had read in a women's magazine that women shouldn't get treated for menopause anymore because it causes cancer.

Poor Mary. She, like countless others, is a victim of misinformation. Let's discuss the truth about Mary's condition, which is a form of hormone imbalance known as *estrogen dominance.*

ROLE OF ESTROGEN

The subject of the hormone, estrogen, is complex because estrogen imbalance—whether too high or too low—can result in many distressing physical and mental symptoms and contribute to chronic illness or premature death. This fascinating hormone plays many important roles in the health of women and men and is best known for being the *feminization* hormone. Estrogen, in a role analogous to that of testosterone in males, is responsible for development of breasts and the components of the female reproductive system—the vagina, uterus (womb), and fallopian tubes; bone growth; and body fat distribution. It is also important in skin softness, brain function, and osteoporosis prevention. Estrogen creates little girls, helps them morph into women, and then causes many of them problems when it and its partner progesterone's levels decrease during the various stages of menopause.

Stages of Menopause

Comprehending the stages of menopause requires a basic understanding of the female sex hormones, estrogen and progesterone, and the physiologic changes that occur when their levels change. Menopause is a set of physical and mental changes women experience as a result of decreased production of estrogen and progesterone by the ovaries. Experts differ when classifying menopause, but most agree it's easiest to think of menopause as having four stages.

Stage 1: *Premenopause*: This is an easy one, and it really doesn't have anything to do with menopause. "Pre" means "before" so premenopause means "the time period before menopause". This is the time period before estrogen and progesterone begin to decline. Because menopause-inducing hormone declines have not yet begun, by definition women do not and cannot experience menopausal symptoms during premenopause because menopause has not yet begun; it does not begin until the next stage known as *perimenopause*. This does not eliminate the possibility of imbalances in either of the sex hormones during this time. Rather, it means that if they ARE imbalanced, it is NOT a result of menopause.

Stage 2: *Perimenopause*: Again, there's no reason to make a simple thing difficult. "Peri" means "around", so if you think about words like "perimeter" or "periscope" you'll realize that both of these terms imply "encircling" or "going around" things. Think of perimenopause as the time period when menopause starts and continues until the woman has not had a menstrual period for twelve contiguous months. Onset varies, but for most women, perimenopause occurs in the early to mid-forties.

<u>Stage 3</u>: *Menopause*: This is also easy to remember because it has a clear-cut scientific definition. Menopause is said to have occurred when a woman of menopausal age has gone twelve consecutive months without a menstrual period. Average age of menopause is fifty.

Please note that a related definition is *surgical menopause*. Surgical menopause is menopause that occurs as a result of undergoing hysterectomy.

There are two types of hysterectomies and both result in surgical menopause. A *complete hysterectomy* [Figure 1 below] is removal of both the uterus and the cervix. The *cervix* is the bottom section of the uterus and is the part of the body involved in *Pap smears*—the extremely effective test performed to identify early cervical cancer so it can be removed before it spreads and causes severe illness or death. Some complete hysterectomies include removal of the ovaries and the fallopian tubes [Figure 2 below]. This additional procedure is called a *bilateral salpingoophorectomy*, or BSO. This type of surgery causes immediate and rapid declines in estrogen and progesterone that result in nearly instant menopause. This makes sense when you consider that in this procedure the ovaries—the organs that produce estrogen and progesterone—are removed and they are not removed in a hysterectomy without BSO. A *partial hysterectomy* (Figure 3) differs from a complete hysterectomy in that it involves removal of the uterus, but the cervix is not removed. The rate of onset of menopause in women undergoing this procedure is rapid, but not as rapid as that seen in women who have also had their ovaries removed.

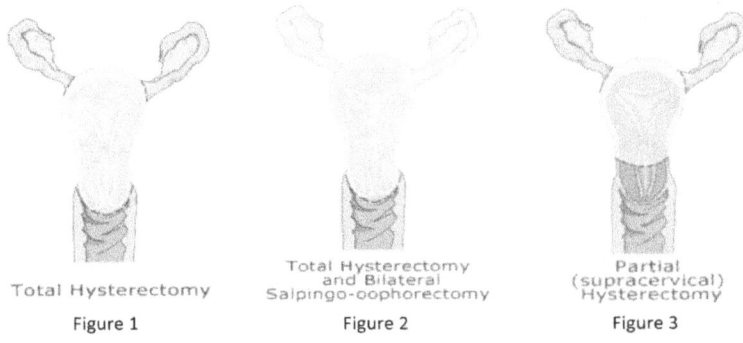

Total Hysterectomy

Figure 1

Total Hysterectomy
and Bilateral
Salpingo-oophorectomy

Figure 2

Partial
(supracervical)
Hysterectomy

Figure 3

SYMPTOMS OF ESTROGEN IMBALANCE

There are two classifications of estrogen imbalance. When estrogen levels are too high, or are high relative to its counterpart hormone, progesterone this hormonal state is called *estrogen predominance*. When estrogen levels are too low, or are low relative to progesterone this results in *estrogen deficiency*. Again, think back to our teeter-totter example when envisioning maintaining balance between these two critically important hormones. From a progesterone point of view, estrogen predominance is viewed as *progesterone deficiency,* and estrogen deficiency as *progesterone predominance*. Estrogen and progesterone require each other's presence in order to function well, and problems result when one of them gains the upper hand.

Please use the table below to help you better understand estrogen imbalance. Likewise, another aid that should help you better understand the sex hormones would be comparing the symptoms in the Estrogen Symptoms Table with the symptoms seen in the Andropause Symptoms Table found in the testosterone chapter. The parallels between imbalances of these two sex hormones noted for their powerful effects on the two sexes are remarkable.

Results of Estrogen Predominance	Results of Estrogen Deficiency
Anxiety	Fatigue
Depression	Vaginal dryness
Breast tenderness	Painful intercourse
Increased risk of breast cancer	Urinary tract infections
Foggy thinking	Hot flushes (flashes)
Fibrocystic breasts	Foggy or muddled thinking
Fatigue	Night sweats
Hair loss	Menstrual irregularity
Irritability	
Memory problems	
Infertility	
Premenstrual syndrome (PMS)	
Uterine cancer	
Uterine fibroids	
Infertility	
Miscarriage	
Decreased libido	
Menstrual irregularity	
Osteoporosis	
Strokes	
Seizures	
Autoimmune disorders	
Thyroid dysfunction	
Premenstrual migraines	
Weight gain—specifically in hips, thighs and belly	

CAUSES OF ESTROGEN IMBALANCE

There are many causes of estrogen deficiency, the most common of which is menopause. Other causes include excessive exercise leading to low body fat, hysterectomy, autoimmune disorders, diseases of the ovaries or adrenal glands, and hypothyroidism, among others. Also included on this list would be poor diet, lack of exercise, and anything causing a relative deficiency of estrogen in relation to progesterone.

DIAGNOSING ESTROGEN IMBALANCE

The female body makes three types of estrogens, and their levels vary throughout a woman's life. Knowing the basic differences between these three forms of estrogen is important because it helps you decide which estrogen

58

product you should use if you choose to begin estrogen HRT.

One form, *estradiol,* is the United States' most widely prescribed treatment for menopausal symptoms. It is converted by the body into *estriol* and *estrone.* Estradiol levels decline greatly after menopause, but remain at a relatively constant low level for the rest of a woman's life.

Estrone is produced by the ovaries before menopause and by the adrenal glands after menopause. Excess estrone levels are stored in body fat, which can cause hot flashes. It receives little use in hormone replacement therapy due to its extreme *potency* (strength).

Estriol plays its greatest role during pregnancy, with high levels of this hormone usually correlating with likelihood of pregnancy success. Estriol has positive effects on vaginal tissues, making it an effective treatment for vaginal dryness and menopause-related urinary tract infections and irritation symptoms. Also, it has minimal effects on breast tissue, meaning this form of estrogen does not appear to play a role in breast cancer. Unfortunately, estriol does not appear to help prevent osteoporosis.

Xenoestrogens are foreign chemicals that exist in the environment which behave like estrogens in the body. These toxic chemicals affect estrogen levels and interfere with estrogen—progesterone balance. The tip for remembering this definition is that *xeno* means "artificial" or "fake" in Latin. Xenoestrogens are heavy contributors to estrogen imbalance issues, with large numbers of industrial, environmental and household pollutants functioning as xenoestrogens. Likewise, synthetic estrogens such as Premarin, Cenesta, Enjuvia, and other conjugated estrogens produced by pharmaceutical companies that are not bioidentical to those produced by the body are classified as xenoestrogens because they, by not being natural estrogens, are "other", or "xeno".

Again, estrogen imbalance is diagnosed the same way all hormone imbalances are diagnosed. The first step is eliciting symptoms followed by a physical examination. If your symptoms suggest estrogen imbalance, you can quickly and painlessly learn your hormone levels by ordering an easy to use at-home saliva hormone test at *www.myhormones.com*. If you already know you suffer from hormone imbalance, contact the professionals at Fountain of Youth MD to find a doctor that can help restore your hormones to ideal levels and return you to optimal health.

TREATING ESTROGEN IMBALANCE

The first step in treating estrogen imbalance requires knowing its cause. For example, treatment of extremely high estrogen levels caused by ovarian cancer is much different than treating mild hypothyroidism or growth hormone deficiency. Once severe or dangerous causes are eliminated, treatment of the imbalance with bioidentical hormone replacement therapy can begin and is guided by following your symptoms and hormone levels.

Because all medications, including bioidentical hormones, can cause side effects and create other problems, your first step when approaching a hormone imbalance should not involve medications. Most people experiencing hormone-related symptoms are not involved in a wellness routine that includes a healthy diet, regular exercise and stress control. If that is you, before you consider taking BHRT or any other prescription medical treatment you should institute these healthy lifestyle changes. You should only begin BHRT if your symptoms persist after maintaining your healthy lifestyle for a couple of months.

Treatment of estrogen predominance is accomplished by—don't forget estrogen's dance partner!—supplementation with bioidentical progesterone. Remember: estrogen predominance equals progesterone deficiency. Raising the progesterone level should reduce or eliminate the symptoms of estrogen predominance.

Conversely, estrogen deficiency—also known as relative progesterone excess, or progesterone predominance—is treated with bioidentical estrogen. As with all hormone replacement, the "right" dose of whichever treatment used is the dose that relieves your symptoms without causing other problems. Again, lab tests are used to guide treatment, but symptom relief is your most important yardstick for measuring progress.

There are various forms of bioidentical estrogen creams and gels. It doesn't matter which form you use, the one that is right for you is the one that improves your symptoms and your health and causes you the least side effects or other problems. The two types of estrogen creams most frequently prescribed are named according to their components. *Bi-est* contains estriol and estradiol; and *Tri-est* contains estriol, estradiol, and estrone. Because Bi-est does not contain estrone—the type of estrogen associated with hot flushes and worsening of breast cancer in persons who have "estrogen receptor positive" breast cancer—most healthcare providers prefer using Bi-est over Tri-est. Recent studies suggest that estradiol is well absorbed by the body and estriol and estrone are poorly absorbed.

While it can be difficult or impossible to completely eliminate estrogen-progesterone imbalance, there is a simple, easy-to remember way to approach its treatment. This method based on the estrogen: progesterone balancing act says, "If estrogen is low, give estrogen; if progesterone is low, give progesterone; if estrogen is high, give progesterone; if progesterone is high, give estrogen." Therefore, if you are estrogen deficient, you should begin treatment with estrogen cream. Begin at a low dose and maintain regular follow-up visits where your medical provider will use your symptom improvement and lab results to gradually adjust your estrogen dose until you are back in balance. Remaining true to our treatment guidance principles, if your symptoms and labs suggest you to be estrogen dominant, there are two likely causes. One could be taking too high of an estrogen dose. If this is the case, you should stop taking estrogen and the symptoms should resolve. If you are not taking estrogen, then you swing the teeter totter back into balance by taking progesterone. The table below helps illustrate the principles used to guide treatment of the four types of progesterone—estrogen imbalance.

Treating Estrogen—Progesterone Imbalance

Hormone Imbalance	Treatment
Low estrogen	Give estrogen
Low progesterone	Give progesterone
High estrogen	Give progesterone
High progesterone	Give estrogen

Setting the Record Straight on Estrogen

What is it about estrogen that causes it to be surrounded by more myths and legends than Sasquatch or the Loch Ness Monster? The answer is that estrogen—the hormone associated with sex, childbearing, breasts, breastfeeding, menstruation, menopause, and the fair creature whose face launched a thousand ships and caused Adam to plunge into everlasting sin—touches humans emotionally. The fact that estrogen has such a profound effect on the lives of every person on the planet is what allows it to maintain a powerful hold on our minds and spirits. Estrogen is the sweet, eternal sap that flows from Mother Nature's tree. It grants us life and lies close to all our hearts.

That being said, much of what passes for scientific information about estrogen is actually misinformation. Let's line up these commonly held "truths" and set the record straight.

Fact or fiction: A woman who elects to begin HRT for menopause because she had a hysterectomy (doesn't have a uterus) does not need to balance the effects of estrogen with progesterone.

Answer: False. This outdated notion stems from the medical fact that women who have uteruses and are treated with *unopposed estrogen* (estrogen without progesterone) have an increased risk for developing cancer of the uterus due to overstimulation of the uterine lining. Originally, the thinking was that estrogen by itself could cause no harm if there was no uterus to become cancerous. Unfortunately, many women have suffered and died from following this approach because of other possible side effects of unopposed estrogen, including increased risk of stroke, blood clots and some types of breast cancer.

Fact or fiction: *Over the counter* (non-prescription) "estrogens" work as well as synthetic or bioidentical prescription estrogens.

Answer: Unknown. The scientific answer to this question is that the answer cannot be known because these over-the-counter products have not been tested against FDA-approved prescription estrogen replacement therapy.

However, the correct answer is that the question is irrelevant because estrogen is a prescription product and selling it without a prescription is illegal.

Fact or fiction: The Women's Health Initiative proved that estrogen causes breast cancer so menopausal and post-menopausal women should never take it.

Answer: Yes and No and No and Yes. That odd answer obviously requires explanation. The estrogen—breast cancer controversy issue is considered by many healthcare practitioners practicing cutting edge wellness and longevity medicine to be one of the foremost medical questions of our era. The *Women's Health Initiative*, or WHI, was a huge study of hormone replacement with synthetic hormones performed for the purposes of determining whether or not the benefits of HRT outweighed its possible negative consequences. The study followed 16,000 women divided into one of two groups: one received HRT and one did not. The HRT chosen for the study was a combination estrogen/progestin considered to be the standard menopause treatment at that time. This treatment, trade name *PremPro*, is a combination of the synthetic estrogen, Premarin—a product made from female horse urine, and a progestin—the name for the class of synthetic drugs designed to function like progesterone. After five years, the study was stopped prematurely because the patients taking HRT demonstrated increased risks of breast cancer (29%), stroke (41%), and heart disease (26%). The increased risk of breast cancer noted in this study was supported by findings in a similar study using the same synthetic hormones performed in the United Kingdom at the same time.

So what does this mean? It suggests that women prescribed the products taken in these studies are at increased risk of developing breast cancer and some other worrisome medical concerns. However, the findings cannot be extrapolated to definitively state that treatment of menopause with all combinations of any form of estrogen or progesterone—whether synthetic or natural—increases a woman's breast cancer risk or the risks for the other issues noted. To make that leap would be similar to saying, "Because the Titanic sank before reaching its destination, all ships will sink before reaching their destination." To make such a huge leap in judgment would be considered ludicrous by most of us, yet that is what influential members of the scientific community and the media informed the world was the take-home message from the WHI. And this ill-informed and toxic message led to countless numbers of women choosing not to treat their hormone imbalance, resulting in unnecessary suffering and severe medical problems from untreated menopause. To add insult to this injury, the findings of a French study published around the same time that was similar to the WHI but used real (bioidentical) progesterone instead of a synthetic progestin showed that the serious side effect findings of the WHI did not occur when bioidentical hormones were used. As expected, because the French study contained none of the dramatic and alarming findings the media likes to report, this study received little press, so a prime opportunity to extol the safety and effectiveness of bioidentical hormones was squandered.

What's that mean for you? It means that if you do not have a strong family history of breast cancer and your breast exams and mammograms are normal, then it's unlikely that being treated with bioidentical estrogen would increase your risk of developing breast cancer.

<u>Premenstrual Syndrome (PMS)</u>

Premenstrual syndrome (PMS) is the most common complaint of premenopausal women. PMS symptoms occur in the two week period before menstruation and may continue into the first few days of menstruation. Severe PMS occurs in 2.5 to 5 percent of women and mild PMS occurs in up to one-third of women. Some women begin experiencing PMS at the onset of their menstrual cycles, but most don't begin having symptoms until their thirties. There are many possible PMS symptoms, but most sufferers experience a combination of bloating, water retention and resulting weight gain, breast tenderness and lumpiness, headaches, cramps, fatigue, irritability, mood swings, and anxiety. In addition, the temporary emotional instability of women with severe PMS can result in outbursts of anger and rage.

Although no instant cure has been identified, most women find small doses of progesterone help, and will occasionally completely resolve the issue. The reason that complete elimination of PMS with hormone replacement is uncommon is because PMS is a multi-factorial problem that has both physical and emotional components.

Stress is a major contributor to be PMS because stress increases cortisol, which then blocks progesterone from binding at its receptors, making available progesterone less ineffective. Because of this, if you are a PMS sufferer with normal progesterone levels it does not necessarily mean you don't need progesterone replacement. Why? Because in order to get your progesterone to the levels you need for it to be effective you have to raise your progesterone to extra-high levels in order to overcome the blockade of its receptors by cortisol. The relationship between stress and PMS goes two ways. Improvements in PMS symptoms usually help reduce your stress levels; and reducing your stress should help improve your PMS symptoms because this reduces cortisol which should, in turn, decrease your progesterone blockade.

While estrogen issues can cause PMS, *progesterone deficiency* (estrogen dominance) is the most likely cause of PMS symptoms because many of the syndrome's symptoms correlate with estrogen dominance symptoms such as water retention, breast swelling, headaches, mood swings, decreased libido, and sleep disturbance.

Another reason that PMS is difficult to treat is that every women has a unique response to the cycling of her sex hormones. For example, estrogen levels that cause anxiety and bloating in one woman may have little to no effect on another. Or one woman may glide through an *anovulatory* (no egg release) menstrual cycle and experience no symptoms while another woman with identical progesterone and estrogens levels may experience excruciating premenstrual migraines, irritability or frank anger when she doesn't ovulate. In addition, some women find that birth control pills or premenopausal hormone replacement therapy cause them side effects (including PMS), while others feel fine. For these reasons, it's important you get to know your body, and refuse to allow anyone to tell you that what you're experiencing is just a psychiatric or emotional problem and that an antidepressant or anxiety pill will correct your problem. If you have PMS, the primary cause of your problems is hormonal, and correction of your hormone balance is where you should begin treatment.

10

Progesterone

J anie was frustrated and irritable. She had gained fifteen pounds in the past two years, her breasts ached and felt swollen, her once powerful mind now seemed feeble and her memory was shot. It was if someone had lopped off the top of her skull and poured a gallon of molasses onto her brain, rendering it nearly useless. To make things worse, her husband was avoiding her like the plague and her coworkers scattered like field mice at the sound of an owl hoot when she entered the office. She felt quite sure that if she had a dog it would hide behind the couch and growl at her when she entered their once happy home.

What was happening to her, she wondered? Had she contracted some rare disease like Mad Cow or Ebola or Lyme disease, or was this simply a case of a good old fashioned nervous breakdown? And making matters worse was that she wanted desperately to become pregnant, but even with her limited knowledge of science and hormones she knew that someone who hadn't had a menstrual period in four months and whose periods had been irregular for the past two years wasn't likely to conceive.

Happily, Janie, you needn't rush to the pharmacy and ask for the pharmacist's recommendation on the latest treatments for Mad Cow or Ebola. Fortunately, you aren't dying from either of those dread diseases. You are, however, being tossed about in the sea of life because of an imbalance between estrogen and progesterone—in your case it would be progesterone deficiency.

ROLE OF PROGESTERONE

Progesterone is the sex hormone made by the ovaries each month when they release an egg. This hormone plays many important roles in female health and wellness, most of which revolve around its relationship with estrogen. The best known example is the menstrual cycle, where rising estrogen levels cause the lining of the uterus to thicken in preparation for fertilized egg implantation; and when this does not occur, rising progesterone levels that would have assisted with implantation and embryo survival, instead cause the thickened uterine lining to slough off in order to prepare the uterus for the possibility of impregnation during the following month. Imbalances in the relationship between these two hormone levels result in the pain, nausea, bloating, irritability, depression and other symptoms associated with problematic menstrual cycles.

SYMPTOMS OF PROGESTERONE IMBALANCE

Because of its close relationship/codependency with estrogen, progesterone imbalance mirrors that of estrogen imbalance. If you understand one, you understand the other. Again, progesterone deficiency (low progesterone level in relation to estrogen) can be viewed as estrogen dominance and progesterone dominance (high progesterone level in relation to estrogen) can be viewed as estrogen deficiency.

This table contains symptoms of progesterone imbalance. Again, note the parallels between imbalances of the two sex hormones.

70

Results of Progesterone Deficiency	Results of Progesterone Dominance
Anxiety	Fatigue
Depression	Sleepiness
Breast tenderness	Fluid retention
Increased risk of breast cancer	Bloating
Foggy thinking	Libido decrease
Fibrocystic breasts	Depression
Fatigue	Vaginal dryness
Hair loss	Painful intercourse
Sleep difficulty/insomnia	Urinary tract infections
Irritability	Hot flushes (flashes)
Memory problems	Foggy or muddled thinking
Infertility	Night sweats
Premenstrual syndrome (PMS)	Menstrual irregularity
Uterine cancer	Acne
Uterine fibroids	
Infertility	
Fluid retention	
Miscarriage	
Decreased libido	
Heavy menstrual flow during periods	
Menstrual irregularity	
Osteoporosis	
Increased cholesterol	
Migraine headaches	
Heart disease	
Strokes	
Seizures	
Autoimmune disorders	
Thyroid dysfunction	
Premenstrual migraines	
Weight gain—specifically hips, thighs and belly	

CAUSES OF PROGESTERONE IMBALANCE

Although books like this spend a great deal of time discussing the roles that estrogen and progesterone imbalance play in menstrual irregularity, premenstrual and menstrual symptoms, and menopause we must also remember that menstrual concerns and menopause only exist because women's bodies were built to make babies. The hormones that make this possible—estrogen and progesterone—work hand in hand to establish the correct physiological environment that make possible the miracle of fertility and human birth.

Breaking down the scientific name for progesterone into its parts should help you remember what it's supposed to do. First, *pro* means "for" or "with"; second, *gest* means "having to do with pregnancy"; and lastly, *erone* implies the class of molecules known as "steroids", the class name for a large group of hormones that includes the sex hormones. Therefore, progesterone is a steroid-based hormone whose main job is facilitating fertility. Everything else is secondary.

The list of causes of progesterone deficiency, or estrogen predominance, includes high estrogen; little or no exercise; poor diet; *insulin resistance*—a syndrome that means "a lowered response to the hormone insulin"; synthetic medications; chronic stress; and *polycystic ovarian syndrome*—a condition that occurs when eggs that are supposed to release from the ovaries do not migrate to the fallopian tubes. These unreleased eggs end up forming cysts in the ovaries, leading to ovarian dysfunction that results in a group of unpleasant symptoms including infertility, acne, weight gain, and increased body and facial hair. Because polycystic ovarian syndrome's symptoms occur in women, and its symptoms include many of the physical changes that occur in teenage males going through puberty, it is obviously a condition that causes its feminine sufferers great distress.

Because of its extraordinarily deleterious effects on health, insulin resistance deserves further discussion. Persons who develop this condition suffer from a group of symptoms that include overweight/obesity, high blood pressure, cholesterol imbalance, and blood sugar instability. This term has replaced what used to be called *borderline diabetes* and is a pre-diabetic state that significantly increases risks for heart disease, strokes, dementia and numerous other serious medical conditions. Unfortunately, it is becoming alarmingly common in both the US and worldwide due to our modern lifestyles characterized by little to no exercise, sedentary jobs, unhealthy high carbohydrate/low fiber diets, high stress, and hormonal imbalance due to exposure to large numbers of environmental toxins.

The most common causes of high progesterone levels, or progesterone dominance, include pregnancy, ovulation and menopause. Other causes include poor diet, lack of exercise, and exposure to birth control pills or hormone replacement therapy.

DIAGNOSING PROGESTERONE IMBALANCE

In our approach to the diagnosis of progesterone balance we stick to the same simple theme we used with estrogen imbalance: "When you think estrogen, think progesterone; and when you think progesterone, think estrogen". Your symptoms and physical examination will suggest your imbalance/s, and the laboratory results are used to confirm them and help guide your treatment. To find out if you suffer from hormone imbalance go to ***www.myhormones.com*** to order a quick, painless, inexpensive and easy to use at-home saliva hormone test. If you already know you suffer from hormone imbalance, contact the professionals at Fountain of Youth MD to find a doctor that can help restore your hormones to ideal levels and return you to optimal health.

TREATING PROGESTERONE IMBALANCE

Progesterone vs Progestins

The drugs sold by large pharmaceutical companies designed to function as progesterones are not progesterones. This class of synthetic drugs is known as progestins, and because its members are not bioidentical, or biologically the same as the progesterone your body makes, your body will not recognize them as progesterone which can lead to side effect concerns such as those seen in the WHI study discussed in the estrogen chapter. These quasi-progesterones are no more pure human progesterone than quasi-estrogens such as Premarin made from horse urine are pure human estrogens. Understandably, when progesterone or estrogen imbalances require treatment with progesterone, bioidentical progesterone should be used.

Treatment Options

There are a great many progesterone treatment options, but most receive little use because of problems related to ineffectiveness, inconvenience, or the fact that their delivery systems do not result in blood and tissue levels mirroring those naturally produced by the body, a situation that can cause undesirable side effects.

One treatment option is suppositories. These come in vaginal or rectal forms, but are rarely used because of leakage, mess and insertion concerns.

Another treatment option is injections, but very few of us appreciate the pain or hassle associated with injections, so these also receive little use.

Progesterone also comes in nasal sprays, but because of the rapid and irregular blood levels resulting from using this method and the fact that modern medicine still does not know whether or not it is completely safe to blast progesterone into the brain—which is what happens to some of the hormone sprayed into the nose—many healthcare providers are hesitant to prescribe this form of progesterone.

Yet another form is lozenges that are placed under the tongue and allowed to dissolve, but prescriptions of this delivery method remain low because it causes a rapid rise in blood levels followed by a rapid drop, neither of which is the way progesterone behaves in the body. Drops placed under the tongue tend to act like lozenges, resulting in similar blood level problems that result in their receiving little use.

Next on this long list are pills. Unfortunately, because of the way the body metabolizes, or breaks down, pills most of the *bioactive*, or usable, drug never reaches the bloodstream or tissues and is therefore wasted. Because of this, very few progesterone tablet or capsule prescriptions get written.

That leaves a sole survivor and our winner: stuff you rub on your skin that gets absorbed into the bloodstream and goes where the body wants and needs it to go. These creams, gels and oils work well whether they are rubbed on or delivered via a patch.

As with all hormones applied to the skin except testosterone, which should be applied on heavily muscled areas, the best place to apply progesterone is on smooth, thin surfaces with high blood flow such as the inner arms, neck, face or palms of the hands. Progesterone BHRT is most effective when given twice daily (use ½ your prescribed total daily dose given two times per day), but if your schedule will not allow this then it's acceptable to only use it once per day (give the entire prescribed dose at one time).

The principles behind treating progesterone imbalance are simple: The first step in managing any hormone imbalance is non-pharmacological. If you are like most persons suffering from sex hormone imbalance, you aren't involved in a wellness routine including a healthy diet, regular exercise and stress control. If this is the case, you should enter into a one to two month lead-in period where you establish and learn to maintain these healthy lifestyle changes.

Only if your symptoms and laboratory abnormalities persist after these changes should you consider BHRT. If this is the case, you should begin treatment with progesterone cream. Start with a low dose taken twice daily, remain on this dose for one to two months to see if your symptoms and lab results improve, and cautiously raise the dose until you and your healthcare provider agree that you are "dialed in".

Likewise, if your symptoms and labs suggest you are progesterone dominant, the cause determines your treatment. If the cause is that the dose of progesterone you take is too high, stop taking progesterone and the symptoms should improve or go away. If that is not the case, then you know from our simple formula that the way you approach treating progesterone dominance symptoms is supplementation with estrogen. Again, we employ the same maxim based on the estrogen: progesterone balancing act we discussed in the estrogen imbalance treatment section that says "If estrogen is low, give estrogen; if progesterone is low, give progesterone; if estrogen is high, give progesterone; if progesterone is high, give estrogen." Because of its importance and the fact that it can be used to guide the treatment of imbalances of both estrogen and progesterone, the information and table presented in the estrogen chapter is repeated here.

Estrogen—Progesterone Treatment
Guidance Table

Hormone Imbalance	Treatment
Low estrogen	Give estrogen
Low progesterone	Give progesterone
High estrogen	Give progesterone
High progesterone	Give estrogen

ESTROGEN: PROGESTERONE IMBALANCE
SCREEN FOR WOMEN

Which of the following symptoms apply to you? To have your test scored and receive immediate feedback regarding your hormone status, go to *www.myhormones.com* and check the assessment link. Please mark the appropriate box for each symptom. For symptoms that do not apply, please select *None*.

n   None   Mild   Moderate   Severe

1. **Increased facial hair**

   None   Mild   Moderate   Severe

2. **Breast tenderness/swelling**

   None   Mild   Moderate   Severe

3. **Pain: Headache/migraine/low back/muscle ache/joint ache**

   None   Mild   Moderate   Severe

4. **Vaginal dryness/pain/itching**

   None   Mild   Moderate   Severe

5. **Fatigue/lack of energy**

   None   Mild   Moderate   Severe

6. **Decreased concentration/alertness/memory loss**

   None   Mild   Moderate   Severe

7. **Urinary Incontinence**

   None   Mild   Moderate   Severe

8. **Irritability/anger**

   None   Mild   Moderate   Severe

9. **Anxiety**

   ○ None ○ Mild ○ Moderate ○ Severe

10. **Mood Swings**

    ○ None ○ Mild ○ Moderate ○ Severe

11. **Depression**

    ○ None ○ Mild ○ Moderate ○ Severe

12. **Acne or oily skin**

    ○ None ○ Mild ○ Moderate ○ Severe

13. **Decreased libido/low sex drive**

    ○ None ○ Mild ○ Moderate ○ Severe

14. **Hot flashes/night sweats**

    ○ None ○ Mild ○ Moderate ○ Severe

15. **Sleep disturbance**

    ○ None ○ Mild ○ Moderate ○ Severe

16. **Personal risk factors for heart disease**

    ○ None ○ Mild ○ Moderate ○ Severe

17. **Personal risk factors for osteoporosis**

    ○ None ○ Mild ○ Moderate ○ Severe

11

Testosterone

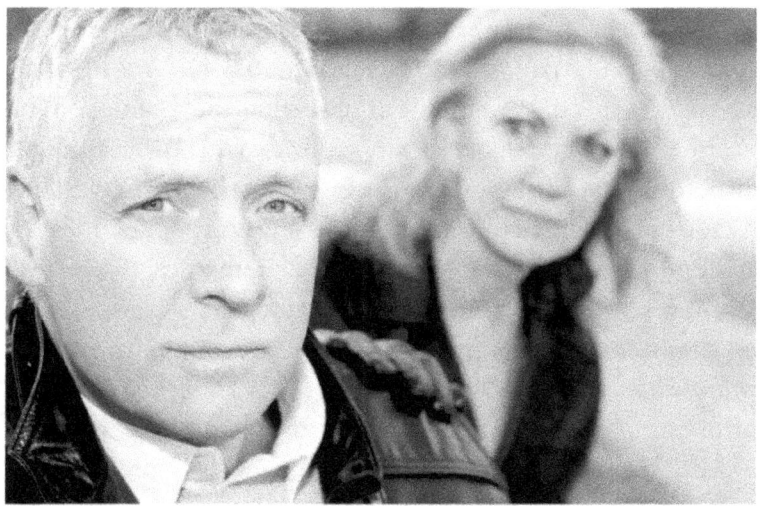

J im threw his sweaty towel onto the locker room floor in disgust. This puzzled Marty, his long-time friend and occasional racquetball opponent, who asked him why he was abusing the poor defenseless towel. Jim snapped irritably at Marty that he was sick and tired of withering away to nothing, and that he couldn't believe he had started growing old in his forties! Marty said he didn't think Jim looked old, so Jim rewarded this kindness with a recommendation that Marty get to his eye doctor soon, because it was obvious to anyone with two eyes that Jim was forty-two going on seventy-three.

The thick-skinned Marty refused to be put off by his friend's surliness, so jokingly asked what he planned to do about his premature aging problem. When Jim asked what he meant, Marty reminded his friend that there are two kinds of people in this world: people that passively allow life to happen to them, and people that assertively grab life by the horns in order to get the most out of it. Jim responded that he understood this, but last he checked nobody had invented a way to stop time. Marty laughed, then told his grumpy friend that he should leave his Neanderthal cave on occasion and pay more attention to recent medical advances—specifically the ones regarding the diagnosis and treatment of age-related hormone imbalance—because he suspected that Jim's aging issues might be treatable. He asked Jim to name all of the things he was experiencing that made him think he was growing old prematurely, and five minutes later Marty informed his friend that it was as clear as the nose on his face that Jim was suffering from *andropause*, which is also known as *male menopause*. He emphasized to his friend that andropause is a medical condition caused by low testosterone and that if he received treatment for it he'd probably be feeling, doing and looking much better within weeks!

ROLE OF TESTOSTERONE

Testosterone, produced by the testicles and adrenal glands in males and the ovaries and adrenal glands in women, plays valuable roles in the health and wellness of both men and women. Although receiving most of its attention for the roles it plays in sexual differentiation and sexual development of males, testosterone balance is critical for men's developing and maintaining muscle bulk, strength, self-esteem, sex drive, mental stability, mental sharpness, memory and concentration, sexual performance, bone strength, and preventing weight gain, strokes, heart attacks, weight gain and diabetes. It plays similar roles in women, and many women are shocked to discover that correcting deficiencies of the hormone most people associate with men usually helps with female sexual desire and sexual difficulty concerns.

TESTOSTERONE DEFICIENCY SYMPTOMS

Testosterone deficiency in males results in a symptom complex known as *testosterone deficiency syndrome*. Also known as *Low T*, this potentially dangerous hormone imbalance, which is the male equivalent of menopause in women, often begins quietly around age thirty and can cause problems in many areas of men's lives.

Symptoms of low testosterone in <u>men</u> include:

- fatigue
- sleep difficulty
- low energy
- decreased self-esteem/self-confidence
- irritability/moodiness
- depression
- anxiety
- muscle loss
- increased exercise recovery time
- body and joint aches
- memory problems
- sexual difficulties
- erectile dysfunction (ED)
- breast pain or enlargement
- weight gain
- hair loss
- testicular atrophy (shrinking)

- increased risk of heart attack, stroke, blood clots, diabetes

Interestingly, the symptoms of testosterone deficiency in <u>women</u> are very similar to those seen in men and include:

- fatigue
- sleep difficulty
- low energy levels
- irritability
- depression
- anxiety
- muscle loss
- increased exercise recovery time
- body and joint aches
- memory difficulties
- sexual difficulties
- breast pain or enlargement
- weight gain/increased abdominal fat
- hair loss
- osteoporosis
- increased risk for heart attack, stroke, blood clots, diabetes

CAUSES OF TESTOSTERONE DEFICIENCY

The primary cause of low testosterone syndrome in males is age-related decrease in testicular function. Other causes include imbalance of other hormones that help regulate testosterone levels. These usually result from problems with the glands that produce them, most notably the pituitary gland or the hypothalamus; cancers or other conditions such as hemochromatosis or autoimmune diseases that invade and replace testicular tissue; testicular trauma or cancer treatment-induced radiation damage to the testicles; and mumps—a viral infection that was once a leading cause of testosterone deficiency but is rarely seen now in the U.S.

DIAGNOSING TESTOSTERONE DEFICIENCY

As discussed previously, diagnosing hormone imbalance is based on symptoms, physical examination and laboratory results. If the symptoms and exam suggest a problem, lab tests help confirm the suspected condition. To accurately interpret testosterone tests, you need to understand how testosterone exists and is utilized in the body.

Total testosterone is the total amount of testosterone in the body. While useful, this number is not the actual amount of testosterone available to the body because it is a combination of the levels of the two types of testosterone: the protein-bound (unavailable testosterone molecules) and protein un-bound (available testosterone molecules). *Protein binding* occurs with all hormones and most body processes, is a critical component in health and wellness, and requires adequate body protein levels. Persons suffering from protein deficiency due to illness, poor diet or other causes may develop protein binding problems that lead to hormone imbalances.

Free testosterone is the amount of testosterone the body can actually use. Because of this, free testosterone is the lab test most healthcare providers rely on most heavily when diagnosing testosterone imbalance and guiding its treatment.

Use this equation to remember the difference between Total testosterone and Free testosterone: *Total Testosterone = Bound* (not free/not usable) + *Unbound* (free/usable)

85

Again, you can quickly and painlessly learn your hormone levels, including total and free testosterone, by ordering an easy to use, at-home saliva hormone test at *www.myhormones.com*. If you already know you suffer from hormone imbalance, contact the professionals at Fountain of Youth MD to find a doctor that can help restore your hormones to ideal levels and return you to optimal health.

TREATING TESTOSTERONE DEFICIENCY

MALES

Historically, doctors have treated men suffering from testosterone deficiency with testosterone injections in their office. Happily, scientific advances in the past twenty-five years have led to additional treatment options. These options, which most patients and medical providers find more convenient, effective and easier to manage, include:

1. Injections: Testosterone injections are given directly into a muscle. In the past, men had to go to their physician's office to receive this treatment. Now, however, men can give themselves these injections at home.

2. Creams and lotions: Patients wishing to avoid injections or who are unable to receive injections for medical or other reasons can receive effective testosterone deficiency treatment with creams or lotions.

3. Sublingual drops: While testosterone has not traditionally been provided in pills or capsules because it would be deactivated during metabolism by the liver, recent advances in the compounding pharmacy industry have resulted in the ability to treat

testosterone deficiency via giving drops absorbed into the tissue under the tongue. This treatment is effective because the hormone is absorbed directly into the bloodstream and bypasses, or avoids, the liver. This leaves the hormone unchanged and usable by the body.

4. Pills and capsules: At the time of this writing some newly-formulated pills and capsules are being prescribed by innovative BHRT providers and compounding pharmacies. This is big news in the BHRT world, as prior attempts to create testosterone pills or capsules that would work well failed because the hormone would be deactivated by liver metabolism. These new products delay absorption of the compound until it has passed far enough down the digestive tract to avoid the product undergoing metabolism by the liver. This allows it to be absorbed into the bloodstream and achieve the blood and tissue levels that help correct testosterone imbalance.

FEMALES

Many women suffering from concerns with muscle mass, energy, or libido or sexual performance issues often find low dose treatment with testosterone cream very helpful. However, those of you who choose to begin testosterone BHRT should remember that the ratio of testosterone in young men to young women is 10:1 and that excessive administration of testosterone to women can result in masculinization symptoms such as weight gain, increase in facial or body hair, thickening of muscles, hair loss, acne, and clitoral enlargement. As a side note, many people are shocked when they hear that testosterone can cause the clitoris to grow. However, this makes sense when you think about the fact that testosterone is the hormone that causes the penis to grow in boys and young men, and the clitoris is the female organ analogous to the penis. And no, gentlemen, unfortunately this potential side effect issue does not occur in men! What you have when you are an adult male is what you have until the end of time. There are no treatments proven to change this physiologic reality.

TESTOSTERONE DEFICIENCY
SCREEN FOR MEN

Which of the following symptoms apply to you? To have your test scored and receive immediate feedback regarding your hormone status, go to ***www.myhormones.com*** and check the assessment link. Please mark the appropriate box for each symptom. For symptoms that do not apply, please select *None*.

1. **Decreased sense of well-being and low self esteem**

    ○ None ○ Mild ○ Moderate ○ Severe ○ Extremely Severe

2. **Joint pains and muscle aches**

    86

    ○ None ○ Mild ○ Moderate ○ Severe ○ Extremely Severe

3. **Excessive sweating**

    ○ None ○ Mild ○ Moderate ○ Severe ○ Extremely Severe

4. **Sleep difficulty**

    ○ None ○ Mild ○ Moderate ○ Severe ○ Extremely Severe

5. **Fatigue**

    ○ None ○ Mild ○ Moderate ○ Severe ○ Extremely Severe

6. **Irritability**

    ○ None ○ Mild ○ Moderate ○ Severe ○ Extremely Severe

7. **Nervousness**

    ○ None ○ Mild ○ Moderate ○ Severe ○ Extremely Severe

8. **Anxiety**

    ○ None ○ Mild ○ Moderate ○ Severe ○ Extremely Severe

9. **Decreased physical vitality**

    ○ None ○ Mild ○ Moderate ○ Severe ○ Extremely Severe

10. **Decrease in muscular strength**

   ○ None ○ Mild ○ Moderate ⦿ Severe ○ Extremely Severe

11. **Depressed mood**

   ○ None ○ Mild ○ Moderate ○ Severe ○ Extremely Severe

12. **Feeling like you have passed your peak**

   ○ None ○ Mild ○ Moderate ○ Severe ○ Extremely Severe

13. **Feeling burnt out, having hit rock-bottom**

   ○ None ○ Mild ○ Moderate ○ Severe ○ Extremely Severe

14. **Decreased beard growth**

   ○ None ○ Mild ○ Moderate ○ Severe ○ Extremely Severe

15. **Decreased sexual performance/frequency**

   ○ None ○ Mild ○ Moderate ○ Severe ○ Extremely Severe

16. **Decreased number of morning erections**

   ○ None ○ Mild ○ Moderate ○ Severe ○ Extremely Severe

17. **Decreased sexual desire/libido**

   ○ None ○ Mild ○ Moderate ○ Severe ○ Extremely Severe

12

Cortisol

M ay Li sat on the park bench and pondered the notion of living the rest of her life feeling like this and didn't like the image that formed in her mind. Being exhausted, frequently ill, sad, nervous, tired, grumpy, and brain dead did not seem like a good strategy for a promising young attorney to employ if she wished to achieve the professional and personal goals she set for herself upon her law school graduation two years ago.

The situation confused her. She knew that most new attorneys had to work long, hard, stressful hours before they reached the coveted prize of partnership in their firm. She also knew that most junior partners are able to withstand this stress and achieve this goal if they also handled the office politics well. She was just as smart and tough as the rest of her colleagues. However, she also knew there was no way she would be able to muster the energy and do the work required to reach the top of the legal mountain feeling like this. Something had to change, and as much as she hated the idea that something might be wrong with her, she picked up the phone and made doctor's appointment.

It took four appointments, eight weeks, a couple of failed treatments, and a battery of expensive tests before the nurse practitioner her insurance company had assigned her to finally announced to May Li that her cortisol testing showed she suffered from adrenal fatigue. The nurse practitioner explained that *adrenal fatigue* was a condition that resulted from problems with cortisol secretion and that cortisol is a hormone produced by small glands located on top of the kidneys called the *adrenal glands*. She explained that *cortisol* was known as the "stress hormone" because it is released by the body in response to stress, and that low levels of this hormone can result from prolonged exposure to stress that results in adrenal gland exhaustion. This happens because the organs that produce cortisol (the adrenal glands) can only tolerate so much demand to produce and release cortisol before these overworked organs tire and begin to fail, resulting in low levels of this critically important hormone. This syndrome leaves it sufferers feeling poorly and renders them chronically ill. And because it affects other organ systems and hormone levels, it increases risks for other diseases and can result in premature death.

ROLE OF CORTISOL

In general, individual hormones have an area of expertise, or physiologic domain, for which they are responsible. Examples of this would include thyroid hormone and metabolism; testosterone and masculinization/reproduction; progesterone/estrogen and feminization/reproduction; and growth hormone's combined role of promoting growth in the young and preventing aging in the old. Cortisol's wheelhouse is stress—specifically responding to stressful situations that require instant focus and energy, such as life-threatening situations.

Adequate cortisol levels are required by many organ systems and body processes such as blood sugar regulation, thyroid function, stress management, protein regulation, mental stability, immunity and illness prevention, and muscle growth. Without adequate supplies of cortisol, all these processes are impaired. Because chronic stress results in overproduction of cortisol, it's easy to see that if you live in a pressure-cooker existence and do not manage your stress well, your adrenal glands will overdo it and you'll enter a high-cortisol state that can result in "burnout" of your adrenal glands—a very instructional term that describes what happens with these physiologic cortisol hormone factories can no longer keep up with the excessive demand placed upon them.

SYMPTOMS OF CORTISOL IMBALANCE

When you read the symptoms of cortisol imbalance below, you will probably find yourself thinking that most of the signs and symptoms of the various hormone imbalances discussed in this book are similar. The fact that they're nearly all the same should help you understand why many hormone balances go unrecognized, why it can sometimes take months and years before a determined healthcare provider finally identifies an imbalance, and why most of today's progressive healthcare providers treating hormone imbalance have their patients undergo a comprehensive, gender-specific laboratory examination that evaluates all of the major hormones.

Most of you reading this book that suffer from cortisol imbalance will be cortisol-deficient. Signs and symptoms of chronic cortisol deficiency (adrenal fatigue) are fatigue, sluggishness, weight gain, bone and muscle loss, depression, anxiety, feeling tired but wired, foggy thinking, and irritability.

Overproduction of cortisol, or high cortisol levels, is another common hormone imbalance. Also known as *hypercorticism*, this imbalance results from cortisol overproduction by the adrenal glands caused by chronic stress as previously described and diseases of the adrenal glands or the pituitary gland. Symptoms of chronically elevated cortisol levels include weight gain, thin/fragile skin, osteoporosis, high blood pressure, blood sugar instability, increased facial hair on females, reduced ability to fight infection, and depression, among others. If this state is caused naturally by irregularities or diseases within the body it is called *Cushing's disease*; it is called *Cushing's syndrome* if it is caused by medical interventions such as administration of cortisol-type medications such as prednisone, hydrocortisone, dexamethasone, etc.

CAUSES OF CORTISOL IMBALANCE

Again, cortisol imbalance is either caused by disease processes that affect cortisol production by the adrenal glands or by medications such as the glucocorticoids (i.e., prednisone, hydrocortisone, cortisone, etc.). Severe, chronically low cortisol states result in *Addison's disease*, a permanent and debilitating medical condition requiring lifelong corticosteroid replacement. Also, Cushingoid states such as Cushing's disease and Cushing's syndrome that result from longstanding elevated cortisol levels are very detrimental to overall health and require identification and correction of the cause.

DIAGNOSING CORTISOL IMBALANCE

As always, the step-by-step process of diagnosing a hormone imbalance is (1) gather the symptoms (2) perform the physical examination then (3) check the hormone levels. If all three suggest a specific hormone abnormality, then, and only then is it pursued. Find out if you suffer from hormone imbalance, including your cortisol level, by going to ***www.myhormones.com*** to order a quick, painless, inexpensive and easy to use at-home saliva hormone test. If you already know you suffer from hormone imbalance,

94

contact the professionals at Fountain of Youth MD to find a doctor that can help restore your hormones to ideal levels and return you to optimal health.

TREATING CORTISOL IMBALANCE

Barring laboratory findings suggesting a severe or life-threatening cortisol imbalance, the first steps towards correcting cortisol imbalance are taking time to make lifestyle adjustments such as improving nutrition and exercise. If you are identified as suffering from cortisol excess (high cortisol) you should be managed by an endocrinologist (hormone specialist) because of the numerous potentially severe causes and consequences of this condition. Likewise, if you are found to suffer from a long-standing cortisol-deficient state you should also be evaluated by an endocrinologist. Most persons respond well to treatment with cortisol, but must be closely monitored in order to prevent complications such as Cushing's syndrome, diabetes, recurrent illness or high blood pressure.

Cortisol vs Cortisone and Legal vs Illegal Steroids

Most non-medical people find themselves confused by drugs and drug classifications whose scientific names sound alike. One question/issue that is important for readers wishing to understand hormone imbalance and its treatment is whether prednisone is a "steroid" and if it is one of the drugs that athletes take for performance enhancement that receives so much media coverage. The answer to this question is that there are different kinds of steroids. "Steroids" are chemicals that possess the same basic molecular structure. Groups of drugs with similar chemical structures are called *drug classes*, and there are two major classes that fall under the heading of steroid.

One class, or group of steroids, is called the *corticosteroids*. There are two divisions within the corticosteroid class.

1) *Glucocorticoids*. Examples of glucocorticoids include prednisone, hydrocortisone, cortisone and other compounds used to treat a wide variety of conditions including allergic, autoimmune, and inflammatory conditions, among others. It's likely that most of you know people who receive "cortisone shots" from time to time. Such an injection would contain a glucocorticoid such as triamcinolone or dexamethasone. Drugs in this class are not used by athletes for performance enhancement and there are no legal or criminal issues related to their prescription.

2) *Mineralocorticoids*. Aldosterone is an example of a mineralocorticoid. These compounds play important roles in salt and water balance in the body and, like the glucocorticoids, are not used by bodybuilders or athletes for purposes of performance enhancement.

Another steroid class is comprised of the *sex hormones* discussed in this book: estrogen, progesterone, and the *androgens*. Members of the androgen class, also known as *anabolic steroids*, are drugs that athletes and body builders use to build muscle and improve athletic performance. A member of the androgen class with which you are now very familiar is testosterone. If used appropriately, there are no legal, moral or other concerns associated with testosterone prescription and use. However, use of other androgens such as nandrolone, oxandrolone, oxabolone, apoptone, and other "muscle builders" is considered medically acceptable (legal) only in rare circumstances, and their inappropriate prescription and use can result in criminal penalties for the provider and the user.

13

DHEA

S ix months after beginning treatment for testosterone deficiency Alan was much improved, but neither Alan or his doctor were completely satisfied with his progress because he still experienced intermittent fatigue and was frustrated at the lack of progress he had made regarding his strength and musculature. Also, his sex drive, while improved still wasn't as strong as he or his wife thought it should be.

His physician suggested that, instead of raising Brad's testosterone dose again they should consider starting him on DHEA. When Brad asked him to explain his recommendation, the doctor explained that raising DHEA levels usually raises testosterone levels because DHEA is a hormone involved in testosterone production.

Happily, at Brad's follow-up visit two months later he reported that the previous symptoms were much improved and his lab testing showed that his total testosterone, free testosterone, and DHEA levels were all normal.

ROLE OF DHEA

Dehydroepiandrosterone, or DHEA, is a hormone made by the adrenal glands that is involved in the production of many other hormones, including the sex hormones. Known as the "Mother Hormone" because of its role in producing so many of the body's hormones, it is unique in that it doesn't have many direct effects on the body, but when DHEA levels are low it can cause other hormone imbalances. DHEA imbalance can indirectly cause significant problems for both men and women because low levels of DHEA can result in decreased levels of estrogen, progesterone, testosterone and cortisol. Like growth hormone, its levels begin falling in most people around age thirty and by age sixty many people suffer from severe DHEA deficiency.

SYMPTOMS OF DHEA IMBALANCE

DHEA deficiency is fairly common and high levels of DHEA are rarely seen. When DHEA toxicity occurs, it is almost always due to an adrenal gland tumor. Women with elevated DHEA levels usually present with *masculinization* symptoms (physical changes associated with being male) such as deepening voice, increased facial hair, decreased breast size, acne, clitoral enlargement, enlargement of the Adam's apple, and increased musculature. Men with high DHEA levels present with exaggeration of these same attributes they already possess.

General DHEA deficiency symptoms include fatigue, decreased sex drive, decreased musculature, depression, anxiety, hair loss, as well as increased risk for heart disease, stroke and memory difficulty.

CAUSES OF DHEA IMBALANCE

Most cases of DHEA deficiency are due to decreased age-related production of the hormone by the adrenal glands. Other causes are our usual suspects, poor diet and lack of exercise, as well as diseases or medical conditions affecting the adrenal glands such as cancer, autoimmune disease, and adrenal fatigue, among others.

DIAGNOSING DHEA IMBALANCE

DHEA level testing is included on most anti-aging laboratory panels. The test used is called DHEA-S, which stands for *Dehydroepiandrosterone Sulfate*. Find out if you suffer from hormone imbalance, including your DHEA-S level, by going to ***www.myhormones.com*** to order a quick, painless, inexpensive and easy to use at-home saliva hormone test. If you already know you suffer from hormone imbalance, contact the professionals at Fountain of Youth MD to find a doctor that can help restore your hormones to ideal levels and return you to optimal health.

TREATING DHEA IMBALANCE

Treatment of DHEA imbalance differs from that of most other hormone imbalances. As with hyperthyroidism, persons diagnosed with high DHEA levels may be suffering from cancer or other serious conditions and should be referred to an endocrinologist.

Treatment of DHEA deficiency also differs from many of the other hormone imbalances discussed in this book because it can be accomplished with either compounded bioidentical products or with over the counter supplements, the most effective of which is 7-keto DHEA. As you well know by now, bioidentical products created by high quality compounding pharmacies are preferred treatments because of their natural properties that lead to better clinical outcomes.

14

Growth Hormone

I t's just not fair, thought the woman as she trudged through her exercises at the senior center. My husband and I worked hard to be able to have a comfortable retirement and live in a nice place. We're surrounded by nice people and they've got enough activities and things to do here to prevent any possibility of us getting bored, even if one of us should pass on. All that's wonderful, but I'm only 66 and feel like I'm 100. And I don't feel like doing any of it!

Unbeknownst to Madeleine, had she taken her concerns to a physician knowledgeable about hormone imbalance she would have been identified with growth hormone deficiency and offered treatment that would not only have helped put the "pep back in her step", but would likely have helped improve her skin, hair, muscle tone, self-confidence, physical endurance and mood, as well as helping prevent osteoporosis, heart disease, dementia and other medical conditions associated with aging.

ROLE OF GROWTH HORMONE

Growth Hormone, commonly known as *HGH* (human growth hormone), is a hormone produced by the pituitary gland in the brain. Growth hormone plays critical roles in growth and development during childhood and teen years, and continues to be of great importance throughout our lives. Its continued presence is necessary to maintain many health functions, including tissue growth, cell reproduction and cell regeneration, which is why HGH has become a mainstay of anti-aging treatment. Declining growth hormone levels associated with aging, known as *adult growth hormone deficiency*, can result in numerous physical and psychological concerns.

In order to prevent confusion, please note the difference between these terms: *Growth hormone* is the name of the hormone produced by the body. *Human Growth Hormone* is the name of one of the drugs used to treat growth hormone deficiencies. This drug goes by the acronym of *HGH*.

SYMPTOMS OF GROWTH HORMONE DEFICIENCY

Symptoms of growth hormone deficiency can be remembered by envisioning the aging process and thinking about the differences between a robust, 30 year-old male in the prime of his life and a withered 90 year-old man who lives in a nursing home. Likewise, results of growth hormone deficiency in females can be envisioned by comparing a smooth-skinned, lithe 25 year-old mother of two children with a balding, decrepit elderly woman with a dowager's hump that resulted from osteoporosis.

SYMPTOMS OF GROWTH HORMONE DEFICIENCY	
Increased body fat	Low HDL (good) cholesterol
Decreased muscle mass	Poor immune system function
Decreased bone density	Poor cardiovascular health
Low self-esteem	Muscle soreness
Wrinkles	Atherosclerosis
Low energy	Depression
Decreased strength	Anxiety
Poor skin tone/elasticity	Increased hospitalization rates
Poor sexual function	Poor exercise tolerance
Decreased organ function	Poor cognition/memory
Low libido	Weight gain
Poor self-confidence	

CAUSES OF GROWTH HORMONE DEFICIENCY

Growth hormone naturally starts falling at around age thirty and steadily continues throughout the rest of our lives. Textbooks and other scientific articles written by conservative physicians who do not support treating growth hormone deficiency for cosmetic and quality of life improvement reasons state that the most common cause of growth hormone deficiency in adults is pituitary tumors. In actuality, there are many people who have both low to low-normal IGF-1 levels and symptoms of growth hormone deficiency caused by aging that would benefit from growth hormone replacement. Other than cancer, causes of adult growth hormone deficiency include conditions and diseases that affect the pituitary gland such as autoimmune diseases, brain radiation for cancer, head injuries, and toxins.

DIAGNOSING GROWTH HORMONE DEFICIENCY

The laboratory test used to confirm growth hormone deficiency is called *insulin-type growth factor-1*. Also known as *IGF-1*, findings of low or low-normal levels of this test in persons with symptoms consistent with growth hormone deficiency justify consideration of growth hormone replacement in persons without disqualifying conditions.

TREATING GROWTH HORMONE DEFICIENCY

Recent surges in demand for growth hormone have been fueled by countless stories of famous actors, actresses and other high profile individuals who have used HGH to remain and act young in order to further their careers using this fountain of youth hormone. The increased numbers of growth hormone prescriptions combined with pressure from influential physician authority figures has led to increased governmental oversight of its prescribing. These hyper-conservative members of organized medicine have

103

demanded oversight of HGH prescriptions because they are indignant that a product traditionally used only to treat children or other people with "real medical problems" such as stunted growth in children and other growth hormone-related growth issues caused by pituitary disease is now being used for what they deem *cosmetic*, or unnecessary purposes. They are also concerned with the possible significant side effect problems that can occur if the drug is used in excessive doses for a prolonged period of time. These curmudgeons are correct when they accuse the drug of being used for cosmetic reasons—reasons such as improving wrinkled and sagging skin, facial musculature, better hair quality, body musculature, and reducing unhealthy body fat—however, they choose to overlook the fact that the most important benefits of receiving treatment with this drug that our body produces naturally is that it helps middle aged and older people who suffer from fatigue, weakness, depression, low self-esteem, anxiety, and it also decreases the likelihood of their developing one or more of the numerous significant medical conditions and diseases known to shorten or contribute to poor quality of life. At the risk of sounding sardonic, what's wrong with a doctor providing a patient a non-addictive product that helps him or her avoid chronic illness, feel better, look better, live longer, and enjoy a better quality of life?

Controversy has surrounded the use of growth hormone because of the "cosmetic issue", questions regarding the treatment's effectiveness, and safety concerns. HGH's use as an anti-aging therapy (treating adult growth hormone deficiency) began in 1990 after Daniel Rudman published a study in the *New England Journal of Medicine* that documented the effectiveness of HGH. The study divided 21 male test subjects between the ages of 60 and 80 who had low IGF-1 levels (the laboratory indicator of growth hormone level) into two groups: 12 received HGH and 9 received placebo (fake drug).

The results of the 6-month study revealed that study subjects who received real HGH injections experienced increases in lean muscle mass, decreases in adipose (fat) tissue, increases in vertebral bone height, and all were also found to have measurable increases in their HGH levels. The control group (study subjects who received a fake drug [placebo]) did not experience these improvements. Rudman determined that the benefits seen with six months of HGH therapy were equivalent to prevention of 10 to 20 years of aging.

Since Rudman's landmark study, HGH was approved for treatment of adult growth hormone deficiency in 1996, and studies by leading physicians and healthcare professionals worldwide continue to confirm its efficacy. The current consensus among these specialists is that HGH therapy provided in a physician-supervised hormone replacement program is effective and safe, with the notable exception that HGH cannot be prescribed to persons who have cancer. In addition, although there is no hard science that supports this additional restriction, most doctors require their patients be cancer-free for at least five years before they will consider providing them treatment with HGH.

Potential side effects associated with excessive HGH dosing include gigantism, stimulation of cancer cells, carpal tunnel syndrome, lethargy, organ enlargement, high blood pressure, headaches, joint inflammation, glucose intolerance, sleep apnea, tongue thickening, excess perspiration, and acromegaly (skull enlargement).

Adult growth hormone deficiency sufferers have two treatment options. Both are synthetic (not bioidentical). One is injections of *human growth hormone (HGH)* and the other is injections with *Sermorelin*. These two treatments both raise blood and tissue levels of growth hormone in the body, but do so in different ways.

If you use HGH, you receive actual growth hormone. Injections with this compound cause an immediate rise in growth hormone levels. The benefits of selecting HGH as a treatment are that it provides a rapid response and works for people with pituitary gland problems. HGH's potential downside is that its use in excessive doses for a prolonged period of time can cause the side effect issues noted above.

Sermorelin is not growth hormone or HGH, but is an indirect treatment method for raising growth hormone levels. This drug is classified as a *secretagogue* because it stimulates the body to naturally increase growth hormone secretion by the pituitary gland. Because of its mechanism of action, sermorelin is not effective for persons with pituitary disease. Because sermorelin will not cause the body to produce excessive levels of growth hormone, its use is not associated with the side effects that can result from careless HGH prescription and usage. Because of this, sermorelin use is growing and some HGH detractors in the medical community now accept its use as a reasonable treatment for physical and mental declines associated with aging.

15

Conclusion

Thank you for taking the time to increase your knowledge of hormone imbalance. The rapidly developing and exciting area of bioidentical hormone replacement therapy is improving the lives of millions. It is our sincere hope you will become one of them and that reading this book leaves you better prepared to adopt the changes that will help you live a happier, healthier, longer and more satisfying life. For more information and current articles, please visit *www.myhormones.com*.

References

Lee, John R and Hopkins, Virginia. *Dr. John Lee's Hormone Balance Made Simple.* New York, NY: Grand Hatchette Publishing, 2006.

Llewellyn, W. *Anabolics.* Jupiter, FL: Molecular Nutrition, 2011.

Pollycove, R. *The Pocket Idiot's Guide to Bioidentical Hormones.* New York, NY: Penguin Publishing, 2010.

Reiss, U and Zucker, M. *Natural Hormone Balance for Women.* New York, NY: Pocket Books, 2001.

Wright, JL. *Bioidential Hormones Made Easy! Look great! Feel great! Lose weight! Have better sex!* USA: Lulu.com, 2011.

Wright, VW and Morgenthaler, J. *Natural Hormone Replacement For Women Over 45.* Petaluma, CA: Smart Publications 1997.

Index

114

R

rBGH (recombinant bovine growth hormone), 27

Rudman, Daniel, 104-105

S

Sermorelin, 106

   Secretagogue, 106

Sex hormones (See also Progesterone, Estrogen, Testosterone), 13, 14, 40, 55, 57, 67, 70, 72, 96, 97

Somatropin (Growth Hormone), 15

Soy, 21, 24, 25, 27

Steroids, 72, 95, 96

   Corticosteroids, 96

   Glucocorticoids, 94, 96

Stress, 15, 25, 33, 60, 66, 67, 72, 73, 76, 91-94

Subclinical hypothyroidism, 45, 46

Sublingual drops, 86

Syndrome, 19, 21, 30, 66, 67, 72, 83, 84, 92, 94, 95, 105

Synthetic hormone, 21-23, 64

T

T3. See Triiodothyronine

T4. See Thyroxine

Testosterone, 13, 14, 19, 23, 40, 41, 54, 57, 75, 81-88, 92, 96-98

   Free testosterone, 19, 85, 86, 97

   Role, importance, 82, 83

   Total testosterone, 85, 97

Testosterone deficiency syndrome (Low T), 83

Y

Yams, 21, 24, 25

About The Authors

Mark Weis, MD is a veteran primary care physician experienced in a wide variety of clinical and leadership settings including full spectrum rural and metropolitan general practice, urgent care, emergency medicine, and medical consultant to inpatient psychiatric facilities. A national primary care thought leader who has performed numerous high level medical consulting roles for the pharmaceutical industry, Weis has been published in numerous medical journals, participated in a wide array of national continuing medical education projects, and has authored two novels, including the thriller Lead Me Into Temptation. A great believer in giving back to the community, Weis's volunteer activities include local and international medical missions, free clinics, Hospice, and Young Life. Having played significant roles in developing numerous successful medical businesses, including Fountain of Youth MD, Canyon Health, and HealthPrice, Dr. Weis—a featured physician in both 50 Most Positive Doctors in America (1996) and Positive Doctors in America (1999)—now resides in Tucson, Arizona.

Douglas Ginter has over twenty years in the health care industry. A former CEO of an FDA-licensed pharmaceutical manufacturer located in Orange, California, Ginter is CEO of Prescription Headquarters, a compounding pharmacy; Physicians Professional Laboratory, a CLIA certified laboratory; and Physicians Products, a physician's management company. He is also co-creator of the Clearly Beautiful line of products used exclusively by dermatologists and plastic surgeons.

Mr. Ginter is a member of American Academy of Anti-Aging Medicine, American Pharmacists Association, California Pharmacy Association, and the International Academy of Compounding Pharmacists.

www.ingramcontent.com/pod-product-compliance
Lightning Source LLC
Chambersburg PA
CBHW070924290526
45795CB00001B/416